Diana Stobo's
Naked Bliss

NAUGHTY & NUTRITIOUS DAIRY-FREE MILKSHAKES
THAT MAKE YOU FEEL SO GOOD!

BY DIANA STOBO

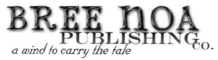
BREE NOA
PUBLISHING CO.
a wind to carry the tale

Published by Bree Noa Publishing Company
P.O. Box 204, West Linn, Oregon 97068
Email: Info@BreeNoa.com Phone: (503) 655-2386

ISBN 978-0-9840892-4-6

Printed and bound in the United States of America on recycled paper with soy-based inks.

By Diana Stobo
35 Miller Ave, #188, Mill Valley, CA 94941
www.DianaStobo.com

Edited by Shawn S. Kipp

Book design by Brooklyn Taylor, www.brooktown.com

Cover photo by Gregg Marks

Food styling by Diana Stobo

Photography by Nancy Dionne, Paul C. Haerr, Gregg Marks, and Diana Stobo

Coconut photo on page 9 courtesy of Luna & Larry's Coconut Bliss

Cover photo: Makeup by Rebecca Mead.
Photo page 159: Makeup by Christina Flach of Pretty Girl Makeup. Photo by Monica Michelle.

Orders for individual copies and bulk orders can be placed with Bree Noa Publishing Company at www.BreeNoa.com.

Dedication

Nature has so much to offer, and I am a consummate produce buyer.

I have a kitchen full of fruits and vegetables and a house full of smoothie drinkers, so the creations never cease around here. Many recipes come out of my kitchen each week, and many people get to taste my Naked creations. There are always those recipes that go unnoticed and are never repeated. And then, there are those recipes that are so ridiculously good, I find myself making them over and over again. When they become really popular amongst my family, friends, and team members, I know they are winners. This is true for many of the Naked Bliss recipes that have often been meal substitutions in my home.

- For my daughter Samantha who loves the Cranberry Chip and Creamy Caramel Swirl milkshakes, I thank you for trying every one of my concoctions, even when you said you weren't "eating tonight."
- For my adored assistant Rebecca who will try everything with gusto as her palate evolves into one that is more accepting. Her favorite is the Garden Bliss, but she seems to love all the Veggie Dreams.
- For my dear friend Ben who loves anything with goji berries and craves the Goji Mojo and Goji Mojo Chip.
- For my sons, Remington and Berkeley, who moan at the sight of yet another tasting only to find themselves delighted and asking for more. Mint Chocolate Chip and Strawberry Recharge are amongst their favorites.
- And for my husband who resists change and yet has changed so much. The man who ate the same thing every day for more than 30 years is now trusting and adventurous and puts his health and nutrition in my hands. He loves the Minty Fudge shake with extra spirulina.

I thank you all for being daring and gracious. I appreciate your discernment and honesty so that I may make each and every recipe a success. I love all the feedback on the recipes I have to offer. They are meant to encourage and delight as we live the Naked lifestyle.

I want to dedicate this book to the people who have trusted me with their health and their palates and who encourage me to keep creating.

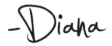

Foreword

Consider yourself in for a treat. You are about to read one of the most healthful books on milkshakes ever published. This book will transform the way you think about desserts and nutrition. Who knew dairy-free ice cream could be so luscious and so good for you?

Diana Stobo is one of the pioneers of the raw food movement. Her first book, *Get Naked Fast!*, inspired me to become even more committed to my own raw food journey. Diana's laid-back and flexible approach to raw foods is a welcome one.

After struggling for years with what to serve my family for a healthy breakfast, I made one of Diana's smoothies. I can honestly say our morning routine has changed because of her book. Instead of waffles or eggs, my kids now request spinach, bananas, and almond milk for breakfast.

Therefore, I was so excited to read *Naked Bliss*. Her scrumptious shakes are amazing *and* good for you; when I drank Diana's Kale Colada shake, I felt like a princess. This book is more than just recipes—it is about creating a blissful experience, right down to adding your GlassDharma straw. Diana includes fantastic information on how to choose seasonal foods and offers numerous little tips to get you juicing and blending fast. *Naked Bliss* shows you how to make delectable and delightfully easy healthful drinks. A sweet indulgence awaits you.

Peace, love & ice cream,

Sandy Henson Corso
Founder, Peaceful Daily, Inc.
Contributor to *The Huffington Post*

Contents

Introduction 2

About Naked Nourishment 3
   How to Find Your Naked Bliss 4
   About Coconut Bliss 10
   There Is No Need to Fuss About Agave 11
   I Scream, You Scream 12
   The Dairy Damage 14

Preparing for Bliss 16
   Blissfully Equipped 18
   Why Eat Seasonal Produce? 21
   Stocking Up for a Blissful Life 23
   Making Nut & Seed Milks 27
   Nuts & Seeds Nutritional Chart 28
   Superfoods 33
   Is Bacteria Really 'Friendly'? 38
   Rejuvelac 39
   Gone Bananas 40
   Fruits With Seeds 42

Recipes
   Fresh & Fruity 43
      To Juice or Not to Juice? 62
   Veggie Dreams 63
      An Apple a Day Keeps the Doctor Away! 82
   Nostalgic Bliss 83
      Citrus 102
   Supercharged Bliss 103
      Raw Chocolate—The Bliss Chemical 122
   Pure Decadence 123
      Getting to Know Your Date 140
   Blissful Fun 141

Diana's Walk-Away Message 159

Recipe Index 160

Introduction

I have to admit, this book happened by sheer convenience. I love ice cream, and to satisfy my cravings I found myself making nut-milk ice creams, coconut ice creams, and every kind of raw, non-dairy ice cream you can think of. They were delicious, but they took time and effort that I found to be above and beyond an everyday treat. Then I stumbled upon a product called Luna & Larry's Coconut Bliss®. I found in it a high-integrity product with minimal processing and no fillers. They were making their coconut ice creams just like I was—with pure coconut milk and agave. *How convenient is that?* I thought, as I quickly stocked up on all their flavors and began my journey into Coconut Bliss®. I would reach into the freezer and pull out a pint and satisfy my sweet tooth with a nibble and a bite. The Naked Coconut flavor is to die for because it is coconut in its natural state. The Vanilla Island is creamy and smooth, and the Dark Chocolate stands out because of the high-quality dark chocolate they use. My absolute favorite is the Cherry Amaretto, as I am a sucker for cherries, so I save that for my alone time.

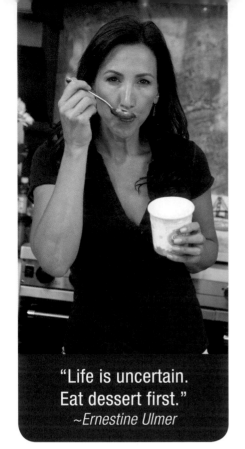

"Life is uncertain.
Eat dessert first."
~Ernestine Ulmer

I love sweets, and creamy sweets are my favorite. When I was a little girl and my family would go out to dinner, I always wanted to order dessert first—a hot fudge sundae, a piece of chocolate layer cake, or some crème brulée. Unfortunately, my parents said that I had to order a meal first. So, I ordered my meal and finished everything on my plate, which was a prerequisite to ordering my favorite dessert. Of course, I was stuffed before my dessert even arrived, but I was determined to have my favorite part of the meal, no matter the consequence. For some of us, dessert satisfies when other options may not.

This book is a love child for dessert lovers like me to adopt sweetness into their Naked Nourishment lifestyle. Now you can have a naughty and nutritious milkshake that makes a satisfying meal. There are so many great ways to use fresh foods, superfoods, and pure nutrition with the yummiest Coconut Bliss non-dairy frozen dessert to create a milkshake that acts as a meal. I'm not saying that you should live on this only, but when you are enjoying Naked Bliss, you are truly living.

About Naked Nourishment

"Naked Nourishment" is a term that I use for any food that does not contain dairy, wheat, sugar, meat, caffeine, or alcohol. These are the six "no's" that I stripped away from my diet as I transformed my life toward better health. Living the Naked Nourishment lifestyle is not restricting or binding in any way, as there are so many excellent and exciting ways to substitute the "no's" from one's diet.

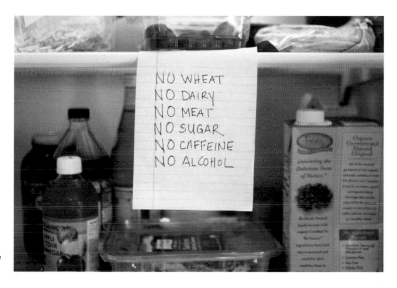

While Naked Nourishment is primarily made up of raw and highly nutritious foods, it is not a truly raw diet. A truly raw diet would not allow some of the alternative sweeteners or sauces that I use, such as maple syrup and agave, which are heated in their processing. Naked Nourishment falls into the category of what is now called a "high-raw" diet. A high-raw diet is one that is made up of 80% or more raw food. Naked Nourishment is not all vegan (which means absolutely NO animal products) because I do use raw wild honey in some of my recipes. Naked Nourishment allows flexibility and creativity with foods so that we are able to enjoy our health and healing process without getting too wrapped up in the details. Most people fret over caloric intake or worry about choosing foods that fall into the guidelines of a set "diet" plan. Being open and creative while fully aware of the foods that are potentially harmful creates a more positive approach to health and, ultimately, a more successful lifestyle. I believe that the "should's and should not's" dictated by outside sources inhibit our own attention to our body's needs. What works for one person may not work for another. Therefore, the term "Naked" allows us to be aware of the foods that are potentially "not working" for us, while stripping away the foods that weigh us down and incorporating more raw foods into our diet.

Instead of looking at fats, carbohydrates, and calories, look for liveliness, nutrients, and minerals.

How to Find Your Naked Bliss

Frequently Asked Questions

Q: Are regular milkshakes really bad for me?

A: Oh yeah, baby. I found this quote in *Men's Health* magazine that painted a pretty serious image and left a huge impact on me. "With the exception of taking shots of melted butter or being hooked up to an IV of rendered bacon fat, there is no quicker way to put on pounds than to tussle with a restaurant-style milk shake." Now for me, there is more to it than the 1,000 calories you would suck down in 5 minutes. It's the quality of the calories, the lack of nutrients, and the very harmful creams laden with syrup and sweeteners that make up this decadent drink. I would never suggest giving up the simple pleasures of life, nor the pure pleasure of decadence, which is why Naked Bliss milkshakes are an exciting substitution for traditional milkshakes in a Naked lifestyle.

Q: Are the Naked Bliss milkshakes healthful?

A: Naked Bliss shakes are a combination of coconut ice cream blended with healthful fresh fruits and vegetables, fresh nut milks, nut butter, super foods, and supplements. Each milkshake is a meal in itself. Sometimes we just feel like having something sweet, and this will relieve you of that desire while filling your body with nutrient-dense goodness.

Q: Are the Naked Bliss milkshakes raw?

A: They are not a 100% raw food product. While most of the ingredients are raw, there are some flavors that are not. For example, maple syrup is not a raw product, and the Luna & Larry Coconut Bliss flavors are not considered a raw product.

If you are not making your own nut or seed milks, then the store-bought product would not be raw, but instead a Naked substitution for dairy.

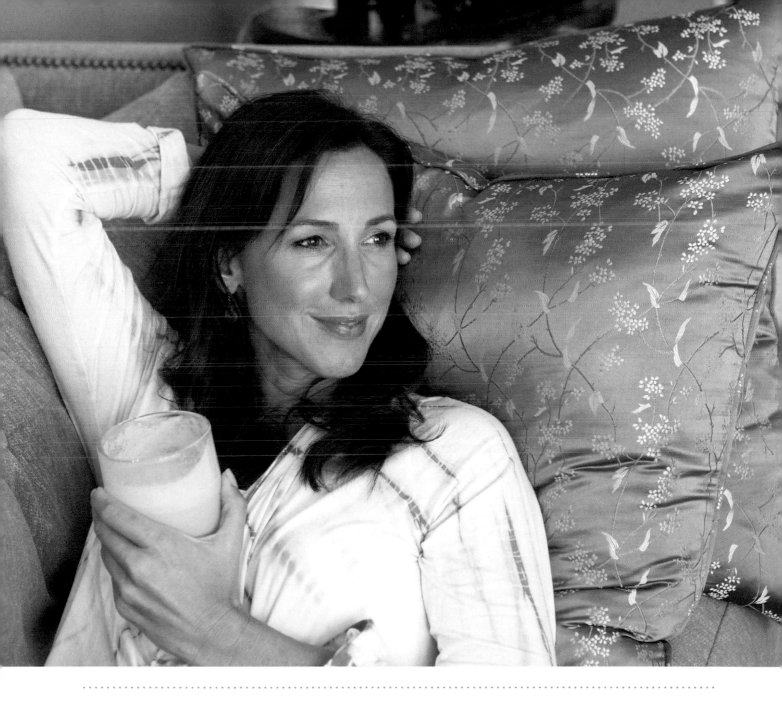

"As I see it, every day you do one of two things: build health or produce disease in yourself."
~ *Adelle Davis*

Q: Why did you choose Coconut Bliss?

A: Luna & Larry's Coconut Bliss dairy-free ice cream is simple. It is the only product that I have seen on the market that has so few ingredients. No preservatives, no fillers, no pretending to be anything but what it is: pure Bliss. Vanilla Island has three basic ingredients:

- Coconut milk—Made fresh on a beautiful, family-owned coconut plantation in Thailand and shipped directly to the Coconut Bliss facility
- Agave nectar—A low-glycemic sweetener made by slightly warming the inulin from the agave plant pod and straining the resulting nectar through a sieve to produce a natural, sweet syrup
- Vanilla—The all-natural goodness of vanilla extract and fresh vanilla beans

Q: Isn't coconut high in fat?

A: Yes, it is very high in good fats that help the body to metabolize. For a long time, coconut was deemed taboo for its high fat content. Over time, research and studies have proven that coconut oil and fats help lower cholesterol levels, promote a healthy heart, and aid in weight loss. This is why coconut is making a huge comeback in the marketplace—everyone wants to get a piece of the once-forbidden fruit.

Q: What about other non-dairy ice creams that contain soy?

A: Soy products in general, while tasting good and providing creaminess and richness, are potentially harmful to your health. Soy is one of the most mucous-forming plants with effects on the body similar to those of meat and dairy products. It is fair to say that if the body responds to the ingestion of a particular food with the production of mucous, then that food may contain a substance that the body recognizes as harmful or toxic. So, I would say avoid soy products when possible.

Q: Is coconut a fruit?

A: The name suggests that it is a nut, but it is in fact botanically a fruit. More specifically, coconut is a drupe, which is a kind of fruit that has a fleshy outer layer. There are other drupes such as apricots, mangos, olives, and almonds. The coconut is actually the largest seed in the world. However, when using loose definitions, the coconut can be all three: a fruit, a nut, and a seed.

Q: Why do my Bliss shakes taste different each time I make them?

A: Nature is perfect in its imperfection, so each individual plant has a slightly different flavor. A cucumber, for example, can range from super sweet to bitter depending on the location, the soil conditions, and the climate in which it was grown. Expect to adjust your shake flavors based on the produce in season.

Q: What if Coconut Bliss isn't right for my digestion?

A: There are many people who are sensitive to coconut or agave and, therefore, need to choose a non-dairy ice cream that works for their bodies. It is easy to use the base of the Naked Bliss recipes without an ice cream. Use nut or seed milk, produce, superfood, spices, and nut- or seed-milk ice cubes as the non-sweetened version of Bliss. It is easy to substitute what works for you and still get the full flavor and nutritional content.

Every recipe is easy to adjust to meet the needs of each body, mind, and spirit.

Q: Can I have a Naked milkshake every day?

A: Yes, you can, depending on your stage of health. When you are eating a Naked Nourishment diet, it is important to stay away from the "know no's" list and incorporate more live food into your diet. Naked Bliss milkshakes are mostly live, raw ingredients that are mixed with a dairy-free ice cream. They are meant to be a treat, when you just feel like having that special something. As long as you eat balanced and mostly fresh produce, you can have your moment of bliss each day. Tune in to your body—just because I say "yes" doesn't mean that it is right for you.

Q: Are Naked Bliss milkshakes high in calories?

A: It depends on the recipe. I would say they average between 300 and 500 calories per serving. If you are considering this as a meal, it really is quite low. But I want to express that if you are eating a diet rich in nutrients, you do not need to count calories—your body will decide when enough is enough.

- -

**Good health is a state of complete physical, mental, and social well being,
and not merely the absence of disease or infirmity.**

Q: How big is a serving?

A: Most recipes make between 12 and 16 ounces. The variation is in the size of the produce. I have found at times that I cannot finish a whole Bliss shake—some are richer than others, and they can be quite filling. They are a pleasure and should be enjoyed as such. Each recipe says 1 to 2 servings to adjust to the individual.

Q: Do I need a Vitamix blender or can I use a regular blender?

A: Any good blender will work just fine. Next to my Vitamix, my ultimate favorite blender was the one I bought at a drug store in college for $15. It had sharp blades and a high-speed option. Some of the fancier blenders promise new technology, but are too slow and can't break down the produce to a smooth consistency. But, if you can afford a Vitamix, it will be the best piece of equipment you have in your kitchen.

Q: If I'm trying to lose weight, should I avoid these shakes until I get to my ideal weight?

A: Let me first say that there is no ideal weight. If you create a number in your head that you believe will make you happy, then you will find yourself "not living" until you get there. Naked Bliss is about pure bliss, eating something decadent and yummy that makes your Naked Nourishment lifestyle more enjoyable. If losing weight is your only goal, then I would sip on Naked Bliss when the mood strikes, but not indulge excessively.

Q: Are Naked Bliss milkshakes alkalizing?

A: Happiness, joy, and laughter are alkalizing. The ingredients in each shake vary, which creates balance. Make sure you really enjoy your shake—sit alone on your patio; enjoy one with a friend; use a spoon, a glass straw, or sip it gently straight from the glass while licking your lips—and you will create a very blissful, pH-balanced environment.

Q: My kids like dairy milkshakes. Will they like Naked milkshakes?

A: They will never know the difference, except that they might notice that their tummy doesn't cramp up after they drink one. The flavors have been tried and tested by my children and their friends. There are some flavors they prefer over others, but they are always excited to have a milkshake when Mommy or Daddy is making it.

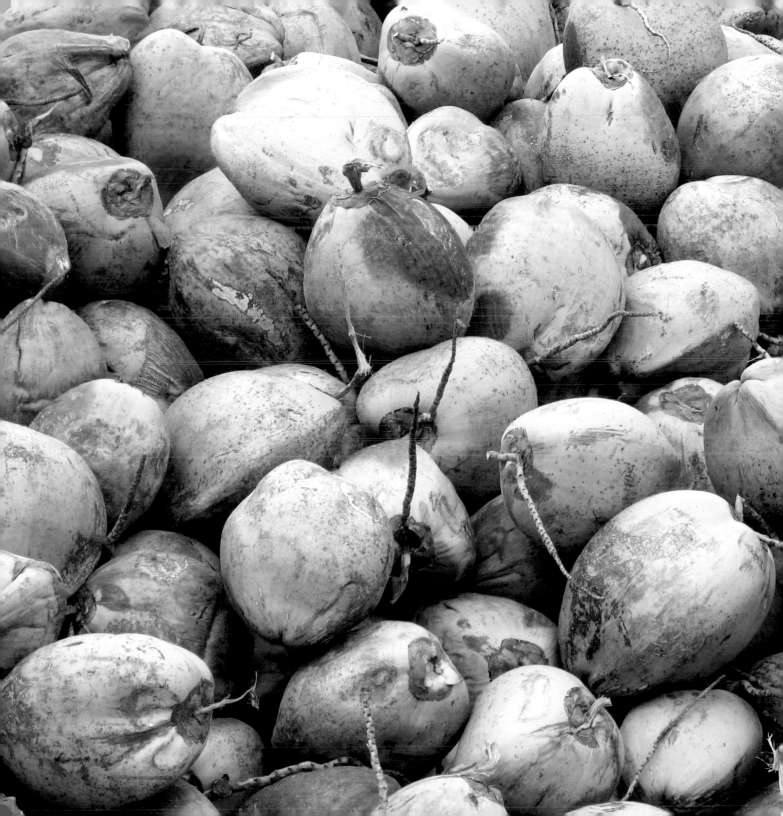

About Coconut Bliss

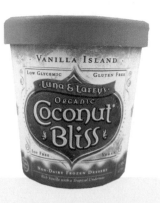

Coconut Bliss is a love story. It's about two people who fell in love over food, and we all know that when love is in the air, creativity flows. Luna and Larry united and set out on a mission to make a high-quality, non-dairy product for their own consumption that fit their vegan lifestyle. Their intention was for good health and great taste. Through experimenting with Thai-inspired coconut-milk ice cream, they discovered a recipe of coconut milk, natural sweeteners, and flavorings that hit the spot. One bite and they knew they had created pure bliss—hence, "Coconut Bliss."

Luna and Larry invited friends to taste their creation and give feedback on this new delight. Everyone was overjoyed and fell in love with Coconut Bliss. It wasn't long before people desired it, craved it, and pleaded to purchase it for their home enjoyment. Local markets and restaurants began asking for it to be sold or served in various locations. Luna and Larry began creating Bliss for more than themselves, and they spread it throughout their hometown of Eugene, Oregon. They were preparing America's favorite food simply pure and natural, without any negative consequence to the body.

> "Coconut Bliss, because of its exceptional taste and creaminess, appeals not just to vegans and lactose-intolerant people, but is winning over people who are dairy ice cream eaters."
>
> ~Larry Kaplowitz, cofounder of Luna & Larry's Coconut Bliss

The business came upon Luna and Larry quickly as it was growing faster than they thought possible. Many facilities offered to produce the coconut ice cream for them to meet the growing demand, and Luna and Larry chose wisely so that they could stand by the integrity of their product without adding stabilizers or fillers.

Coconut Bliss has gained its success, and Luna and Larry have kept true to their desires and their word in creating an all-natural "clean" ice cream that promises pure bliss.

"Coconut Bliss is real food, made of simple ingredients that we found in our kitchen, without fillers or chemical additives, and it tastes great. We continue to make it with love and intention." ~Luna and Larry

There Is No Need to Fuss About Agave ...

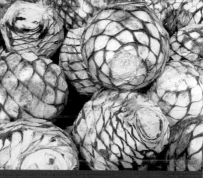

Underneath the spiky tips of the agave plant lies *la piña*. This is where the heart and soul live. The larger *la piña*, the more mature the sugars. Patience equals greatness.

Unless you are drinking it by the cupful. Agave is a concentrated sweetener, used sparingly to create a gentle sweetness that is familiar to most palates. It has recently won the hearts of millions of people for its low-glycemic, non-invasive effects on the human body. It has made a great substitute for processed sugars in many people's diets, and it is being sold everywhere.

Not too long ago an article was written claiming that agave nectar is no better than corn syrup. It said agave is processed similarly to corn syrup and has the same effect on the body as a high-glycemic, high-fructose sweetener. The accusations were more than most could take, stripping people of their joy and sweet pleasure.

My advice to anyone who has sugar sensitivities, and especially diabetes, is to stay away from all sweeteners. But, if you are simply trying to make a healthful substitution for sugar in your Naked lifestyle, then agave nectar can be quite satisfying.

The agave used in Luna & Larry's Coconut Bliss comes from a pristine processing plant in Jalisco, Mexico, where the agave piñas are ground up and sprayed with water to remove the juice. The juice is then gently heated to break down the inulin into fructose, filtered for impurities, and finally evaporated using heat and a vacuum to turn it into a thick, luscious syrup.

The agave plants themselves come from a USDA-certified organic farm where there are no fertilizers, pesticides, herbicides, or even water used to grow them. They are grown in the environment in which they naturally thrive.

So, when you find yourself getting into a conundrum of too much thought and information, take a step back and just listen to your body. How does it respond to agave? Do you get headaches? Heart palpitations? Or do you just get a yummy, blissful satisfaction? Either way, your body will let you know.

I Scream, You Scream ...

We all scream for ice cream! The "great American dessert" has been around since the 13th century, although back then it did not look, taste, or feel the way it does today—sweet, creamy, and smooth. Like most foods, it evolved as our culinary skills, technology, and taste buds evolved. Milkshakes were created much later, long after ice cream was the beloved American food. What started as an alcoholic whiskey drink with a thick eggnog texture soon became a concoction of soda and syrups: chocolate, vanilla, and strawberry. In 1922, a man named Stephen Poplawski invented a cool device: the electric blender, which changed the world as we knew it. This new piece of equipment sparked the imagination of a soda jerk at a Walgreen's in Chicago, Illinois, named Ivar "Pop" Coulson. He added 2 scoops of ice cream to his syrupy sweet concoction. He called it an "old-fashioned malted milk," and it quickly became a popular drink that sparked the launch of malt shops around the country.

Malt shops were the "coffee shops" of their day. They were a social gathering, a place to meet up and hang out, and they were a part of America's youth culture. Many a first kiss and even wedding engagements were made after couples shared a syrupy sip through the dual straws in their old-fashioned malted.

Recognizing the community-building that sparked from this delicious creation, school systems began to serve milkshakes in their lunch program. In 1936, Earl Prince invented a milkshake machine called the Multimixer that could automatically dispense milkshakes at a rapid rate, thanks to the invention of Freon-cooled refrigerators. I guess you could say milkshakes are a phenomenon of modern technology and love.

The popularity of milkshakes was overwhelming, and all it took was a young Multimixer salesman by the name of Ray Kroc to see that there was big money in this treat. Being the entrepreneur that he was, he bought exclusive rights to the invention. Although the Ray Kroc who began the McDonald's fast-food restaurant chain may not have been into a Naked lifestyle, he certainly knew what people wanted and became very successful in giving it to them.

Milkshakes are part of America. For years, people have enjoyed the frozen, dessert-like beverage. About 2 billion servings are recorded as being sold per year. And that doesn't even account for the homemade ones that families deem a treat. It is such a pleasure to be able to continue the tradition of joy, youth, and community through America's favorite treat, as our health consciousness keeps evolving.

What the Average American Consumes in a Year

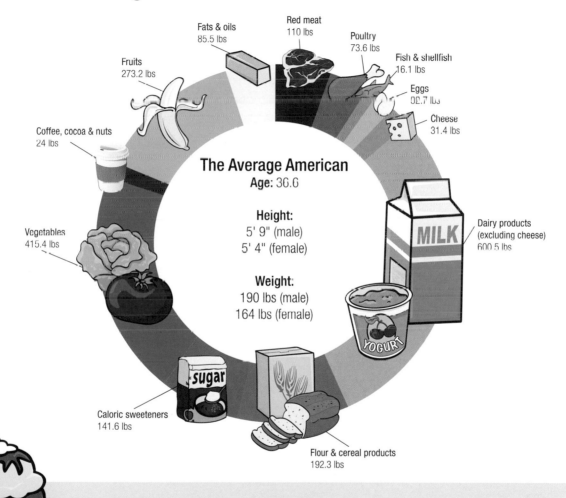

Fats & oils
85.5 lbs

Red meat
110 lbs

Poultry
73.6 lbs

Fish & shellfish
16.1 lbs

Eggs
02.7 lbs

Cheese
31.4 lbs

Fruits
273.2 lbs

Coffee, cocoa & nuts
24 lbs

Vegetables
415.4 lbs

Dairy products
(excluding cheese)
600.5 lbs

The Average American
Age: 36.6

Height:
5' 9" (male)
5' 4" (female)

Weight:
190 lbs (male)
164 lbs (female)

Caloric sweeteners
141.6 lbs

Flour & cereal products
192.3 lbs

Each American consumes about 24 pounds of ice cream each year. That is 24 pounds of pasteurized and homogenized dairy, sugary syrups, processed sugar, artificial flavors and enhancers, stabilizers, and preservatives, which the body does not know how to process.

The Dairy Damage

Dairy is consumed in mass quantity in America. The average American consumes 24 pounds of ice cream every year. I know that may seem impossible, but a year is a long time, and if you really think about how easy it is to sneak a scoop here and a nibble there, it adds up quickly. And that does not even include milk, cheese, and butter. We are a nation with a high disease rate, one being a huge increase in osteoporosis. Most medical doctors, with the best intention, will encourage you to increase your calcium intake to aid in strengthening your bones. They will suggest eating yogurt, cottage cheese, and, of course, milk. While it is true that dairy does contain calcium, the dairy damage is much greater than the benefits.

Dairy enters the body as an acidic food, throwing the natural pH balance off and triggering the body to neutralize the acidic intruder. The highly alkalizing calcium that is in our bones is the most obvious neutralizer because it quickly absorbs acids. Think of how baking soda might absorb liquid quickly and efficiently. Because our bodies are highly intelligent and know how to heal themselves, they swiftly take action. So, calcium is naturally leached from our bones, the very foundation of our structure. Over time, this bone depletion turns into its given name: osteoporosis.

Nature vs. Nurture

Nature meant for us to consume our mother's milk until we wean from her. As our body matures and stops producing the milk-digesting enzyme lactase, it is letting us know that we no longer have a nutritional need for milk. We are meant to move to Mother Earth for nourishment.

Nurture teaches us to continue the suckling by getting our protein and calcium from other sources, such as cows, goats, and sheep. Even though these are a poor substitute for mama's breast milk, they feed the hungry and keep humans nourished. Animal milk can be produced unnaturally and abundantly without an offspring to feed so that humans may nourish from other animals as nurture dictates.

Know Your Cow

Raw dairy, fresh from the source, has active enzymes that help you digest and assimilate the protein in milk. But unless you live on a farm and get it directly from the cow, goat, or sheep, you are receiving a quart of curiosity. Who is the source of the milk? What is the animal's health condition? How long has the milk been stored before purchase? There are too many variables for me to ever consider consuming it.

Pasteurization and homogenization are processes that have been created to give dairy a longer shelf life, a creamier texture, and a prettier look. Like many of our foods today, milk has been modified for uniformity and convenience. Not a bad idea, until our bodies begin to retaliate. Now, we must ask, what's the point?

Pasteurization is a process of heating foods to a specific temperature that kills all harmful microorganisms and bacteria. This process started when people began contracting illnesses from raw dairy products. A brilliant solution, don't you think? Unfortunately, pasteurization also kills all beneficial enzymes that aid in the digestion of the product.

Homogenization is a treatment that prevents the natural separation of the cream-top layer from the low-fat layer of milk. It's meant to be a beautifying process that creates a more consistent and creamy end result. The process of homogenization is not a pretty picture, however. It is done through high-pressure pumps where the raw milk undergoes extreme turbulence and "cavitation." Hydraulic pumps send shock waves into the milk, creating significant damage to its molecular parts. This is an extremely undesirable phenomenon for a healthy body. I don't know about you, but anything that has gone through scorching temperatures and damaging pumps to appeal to my senses, just lost its appeal.

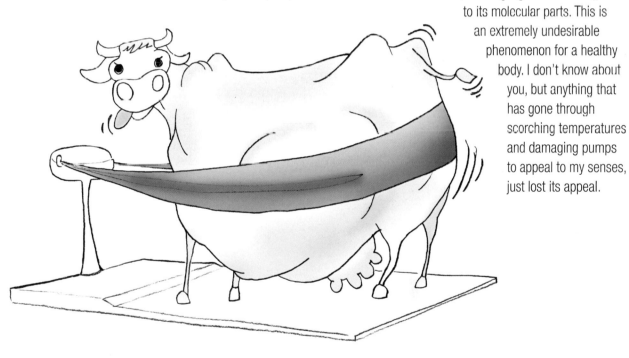

The calcium in dairy is not available to the human body. Most humans stop producing the enzyme lactase that enables us to metabolize lactose, making dairy a foreign substance to our brilliant bodies.

Preparing for Bliss

Preparing for Bliss should be easy once you have found your way to Naked Nourishment. If you have read *Get Naked Fast!,* updated your diet to follow the "know no's" list, and understand the substitutions, you have probably changed your pantry items to foods that nourish the body. I sure hope so, because it will make your road to Bliss that much more joyful. If you haven't, the guidelines below will get you stocked and ready for Naked Bliss.

A dairy-free ice cream is a must. Find one that rocks your world. Whether it is made of almond milk, coconut milk, cashews, or even hemp, I say find the one that makes you happy. I have chosen Luna & Larry's Coconut Bliss as my favorite, and I can tell you that you will not be disappointed if you try it as well. I am a grocery store stalker, and I check out different markets around the world looking for product selection and availability, so I am fully aware that you cannot always find the items that I mention. So be kind to yourself and make the proper changes that are necessary for both ease and delight.

Nut and seed milks are a must in the pantry or refrigerator. They are available in all different kinds of ways: boxed, refrigerated, mixed flavors, or in cream form. You just have to look to see how many different brands are out there. If nuts or seeds cause your body any grief there are also rice milks, oat milks, and multi-grain milks for you to choose from. However, I highly suggest that anybody who loves milky products learn to make their own (for instructions, see p. 27).

Fresh fruits and vegetables are always a must when preparing for a Naked lifestyle. The very foundation of getting Naked is consuming a mostly plant-based diet, with plants as close to their natural state as possible, when possible. Again, I realize that not everyone lives on an island with mineral-rich soil or in a mild climate where crops produce all year long. Therefore, it is important to be creative and experimental. Eat fresh, live, organic produce when you can, and when you can't, supplement with frozen produce and superfoods.

Superfoods are mighty, medicinal foods that are power-packed with nutrients. They come from all over the world and are often available in powder form. Green powders can carry you through those winter months when fresh greens may not be available in abundance. There are also highly nutritive fruit powders that can nourish the body with their antioxidants, vitamins, and minerals. Be courageous—take a chance on the unknown items that may have just been brought to your attention and add some unique superfoods that you may already be using in your routine. In this book, I have just tapped the surface of these powerhouse foods, so I encourage you to dive deeper into learning about what these superfoods have to offer (for more information and a list of superfoods, see pp. 33 to 37).

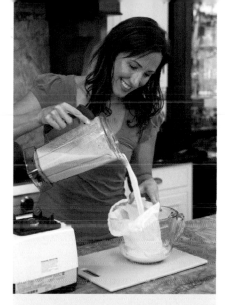

Stock up on your favorite nuts and seeds, get yourself a nut-milk bag, and give it a try (see Making Nut & Seed Milks on p. 27).

Good, sweet additions, like honeys, dates, and yummy juices all at your fingertips, will make for blissful fun. Choose raw, wild honey; find a local bee farmer who may supply you with the finest honey. Dates are available in the fall in northern America, and they can be purchased at a discount in bulk from most online sources or local farmers. The beauty of knowing your dates is that they will keep you satisfied all year long if stored properly. Juice your own juices or buy them from local farms (for more information on purchasing fresh juice, see "To Juice or Not to Juice?" on p. 62).

"I doubt whether the world holds for any one a more soul-stirring surprise than the first adventure with ice cream." ~*Heywood Broun*

Blissfully Equipped

Nut-milk bag

This is such a versatile piece of equipment that you will want to have a few on hand at all times. It is a fine-mesh nylon bag that very thoroughly strains the nut and seed milks for a clean and creamy consistency. It is also excellent as a sprouting bag for sprouting your wheat and rye to make rejuvelac, the probiotic drink I use in many recipes to create a yogurt-like taste. Another great use is if you do not have a juicer but want to make non-pulpy juices. Just blend the fruit or vegetable with water in your blender and pour through the bag to get a delicious juice.

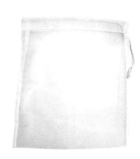

Blender

While it is true that any blender will do, make sure it is the blender that works for you. I strongly advocate purchasing a supersonic blender like the Vitamix®, but not everyone can afford such a luxury, and I don't want that to be a reason for anyone to not move forward into health. My favorite blender of all time is the one I bought for $15 in a local drug store when I entered college 900 years ago. It had a plastic canister, a sharp blade, and a fast motor. I used it for nearly 20 years before I spoiled myself with a Vitamix®.

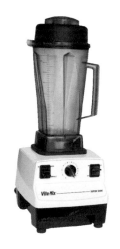

Ice cream paddle

There is no need for a pretty little scooper when making shakes. You want to paddle the Coconut Bliss right out of its container straight into the blender of choice. I'm not even sure I measured most of the ice cream I put into each shake: one paddle meant half a cup, two paddles meant a full cup, and three paddles was a full cup and a half. So, whether you are using a scoop, a spoon, or a paddle, make sure you can get the Bliss out of the container with ease.

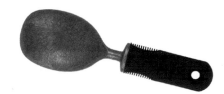

Cold-coffee press

The Hourglass® Coffee System is a fancy device for making a smooth, low-acid coffee concentrate. The beauty of this piece of equipment is that it has a fine filter that ensures a ground free concentrate. You may also use a French coffee press for a similar result, but I believe this piece of equipment works best. And it's very cute, don't you think?

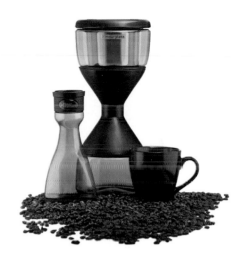

Juicer

I think everyone should have a juicer in the home. All that matters is that you like it. It has to be user friendly and easy to clean or it will be stored deep in the pantry with cobwebs on it. That won't be doing anyone any good. I have found the Green Star®, Solo Star®, and Solo Star II® machines to be my favorites, and I have tried them all. The one thing I know is no matter how much you pay for your juicer, eventually one part will need to be replaced. So, choose one that makes you happy.

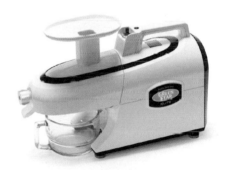

Spice and nut grinder

When adding spices to your Naked Bliss shakes, I think it best to grind them fresh from seed, pod, or leaf. It may have you adjusting the flavors a bit because freshly ground spices are much more robust and flavorful. This is a great piece of equipment because it also grinds nuts, seeds, and even coffee. I use this quite often in my home, and I'm not really a device kind of girl.

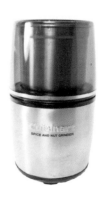

Citrus juicer

I used to hand-juice most of my juices, and it drove everyone crazy. So I got myself an electric juicer to see what I was missing out on, and let me say, a lot! This juicer makes juicing fruits so easy. I buy a big bag of oranges from a farmers' market and spend only a few minutes to juice a quart or two of fresh juice. Sometimes you just have to laugh at how difficult we make things to be.

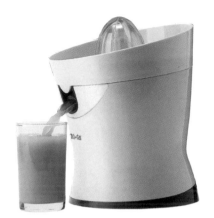

Strainer

A fine-mesh strainer is good for so many things, I just couldn't resist placing it in this book. It's great for the obvious—rinsing of fresh fruits and vegetables—but it is also great for straining your soaked nuts and seeds. It acts as a wonderful sprouting tray when placed over a bowl for overflow, and is a fine sieve for pulpy juice. Have one around the house and you will see how often you use it.

GlassDharma drinking straw

After trying these lovely glass straws, I was smitten. They are beautiful additions to your milkshakes as they come in an array of designs and colors, but they are also practical and useful. If you like sipping from a straw, this is a great alternative to the plastic versions. They are eco-friendly and easily washable.

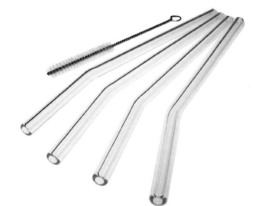

Simple down—life doesn't have to be that hard.

Why Eat Seasonal Produce?

It simply tastes better!

As soon as produce is picked, the nutrients and enzymatic activity begin to decline. It is something we pay little attention to because we are accustomed to having most fruits and vegetables available year round. Most likely we are so pleased to be eating healthfully that we haven't considered how far the produce may have traveled to arrive in our local markets. The non-seasonal produce, even at its finest, is mostly devoid of nutrition by the time we consume it and probably won't add benefit to our bodies. Eating mostly seasonal and local produce, when possible, will ensure maximum nutrients throughout the year.

Seasonal: These are fruits and vegetables that are being grown naturally where the weather conditions are right for their germination and growth. Think of perennials that blossom one time each year as they are waiting for the right environmental circumstances (i.e., heat, light, and moisture) to burst into life. Plants grown in season grow "naturally" and need fewer chemicals and fertilizers. Ultimately, they are the most beneficial to our bodies, the planet, and our lives.

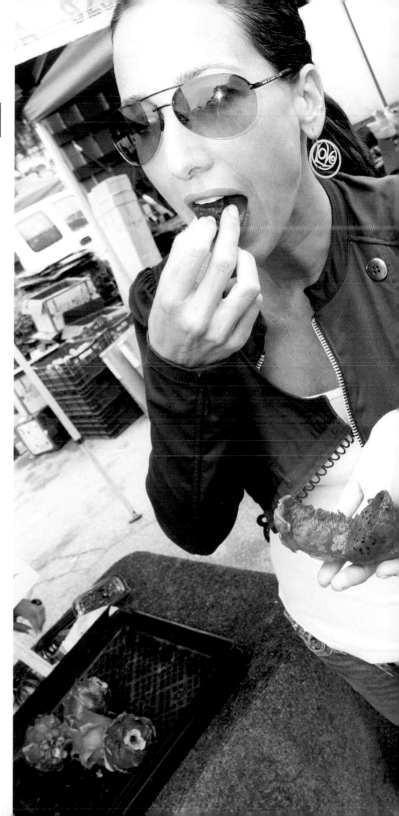

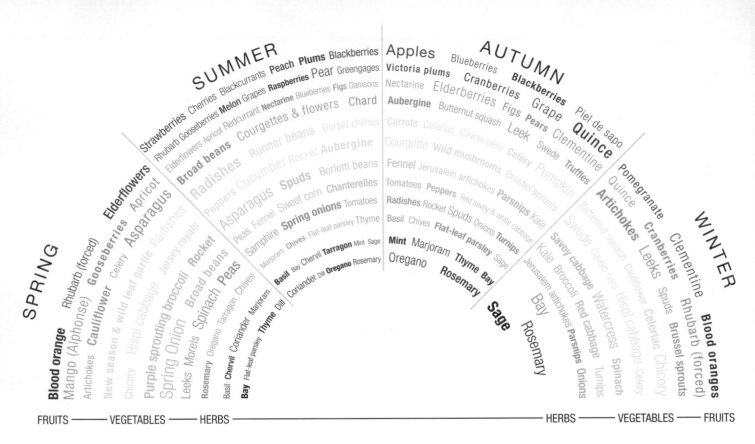

SUMMER

SPRING

AUTUMN

WINTER

Apples

Strawberries Cherries Blackcurrants **Peach Plums** Blackberries
Rhubarb Gooseberries **Melon** Grapes **Raspberries** Pear Greengages
Elderflowers Apricot Redcurrant **Nectarine** Blueberries **Figs** Damsons
Broad beans Courgettes & flowers Chard
Radishes Runner beans Dorset chillies
Peppers Cucumber Rocket **Aubergine**
Asparagus **Spuds** Borlotti beans
Peas Fennel Sweet corn Chanterelles
Samphire **Spring onions** Tomatoes
Marjoram Chives Flat-leaf parsley Thyme
Basil Bay Chervil **Tarragon** Mint Sage
Basil **Chervil** Coriander Marjoram
Rosemary Oregano Tarragon Chives
Bay Flat-leaf parsley **Thyme** Dill
Coriander Dill **Oregano** Rosemary
Oregano
Mint Marjoram
Thyme Bay
Rosemary
Sage

Elderflowers
Gooseberries Apricot
Cauliflower Celery Asparagus
New season & wild leaf garlic Radishes
Chicory Hispi cabbage Jersey royals
Purple sprouting broccoli Rocket
Spring Onion Broad beans
Leeks Morels Spinach **Peas**
Rosemary Oregano Tarragon Chives

Blood orange
Mango (Alphonse)
Artichokes
Rhubarb (forced)

Victoria plums Blueberries
Nectarine Cranberries **Blackberries**
Aubergine Elderberries Figs Grape Piel de sapo
Carrots Celeriac Cavolo nero Leek Pears Clementine **Quince**
Courgette **Wild mushrooms** Celery Swede
Fennel Jerusalem artichokes Brussel sprouts Pumpkin **Truffles**
Tomatoes **Peppers** Red savoy & white cabbage **Parsnips** Kale
Radishes Rocket Spuds Onions **Turnips**
Basil Chives **Flat-leaf parsley** Sage
Bay
Rosemary

Piel de sapo
Pomegranate
Artichokes
Cranberries
Leeks
Blood oranges

Swede
Savoy cabbage Cavolo nero Cauliflower Hispi cabbage **Celeriac** Chicory
Kale Broccoli Red cabbage Turnips
Jerusalem artichokes **Parsnips** Onions
Watercress Spinach Celery
Clementine
Rhubarb (forced)
Brussel sprouts

FRUITS —— VEGETABLES —— HERBS ———————————————————— HERBS —— VEGETABLES —— FRUITS

Non-seasonal: These are plants that are forced to grow in an artificial environment by using extra resources (i.e., heating, bright lights, and pumped water) to make them flourish. Imagine trying to grow wildflowers at the North Pole. Plants grown out of season are rarely organic because of the artificial circumstances. Plants that come from far-away sources are usually grown in developing countries with cheaper resources. Overall, they are not the optimal choice for pure health, but are clearly a fortunate option for versatility and convenience.

To ensure optimal taste, nutrients, and bliss, buy locally and seasonally when possible—you may never go back!

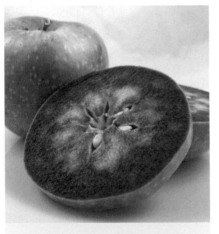

Eating seasonally keeps
you aligned with nature.

Stocking Up for a Blissful Life

Luna & Larry's Coconut Bliss
- Vanilla Island
- Dark Chocolate
- Naked Coconut

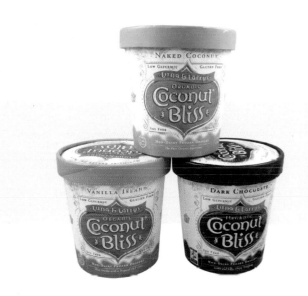

Dairy-Free Milks & Creams
- Pacific Natural Foods Organic Almond and Hazelnut Non-Dairy Beverages
- So Delicious® Coconut Milk Beverage
- Blue Diamond® Almond Breeze® Non-Dairy Beverage
- Tempt™ Hempmilk

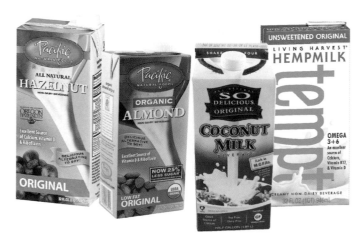

Rejuvelac

- The Rejuvenation Company Rejuvelac

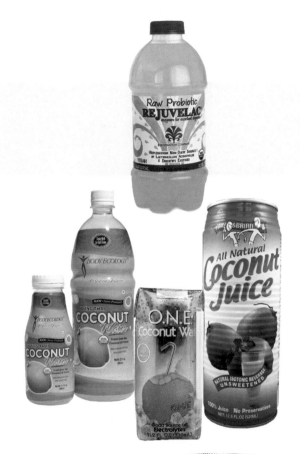

Coconut Water

- O.N.E.™ Coconut Water
- Amy & Brian All Natural Coconut Juice
- Body Ecology™ Coconut Water

Honey/Bee Products

- Really Raw® Honey
- Y.S. Organic Bee Farms Organic Honey and Royal Jelly
- Marshall's Farm Natural Honey
- Wholesome Sweeteners® Fair Trade Certified™ Organic Raw Honey

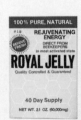

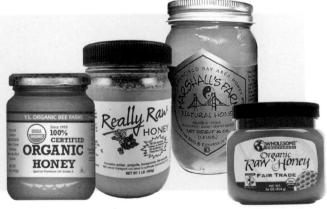

Superfoods

- Earthrise® Spirulina
- Earth Circle Organics raw cacao/raw nibs
- Ojio Raw, Organic Lucuma Powder, Mesquite Pod Meal, Maca Powder, and Cacao Powder
- Royal Himalayan Raw, Organic Gojiberries, Tocos Plus, and Divine Organics Raw Vanilla Powder
- Navitas Naturals Organic Yacon Syrup and Camu Powder
- HealthForce Nutritionals Spirulina Azteca™ and MacaForce™ Maca Powder
- Nutrex Hawaii Spirulina pacifica™
- Maca Magic™ Whole Raw Powder
- Body Ecology™ Frozen Coconut Meat

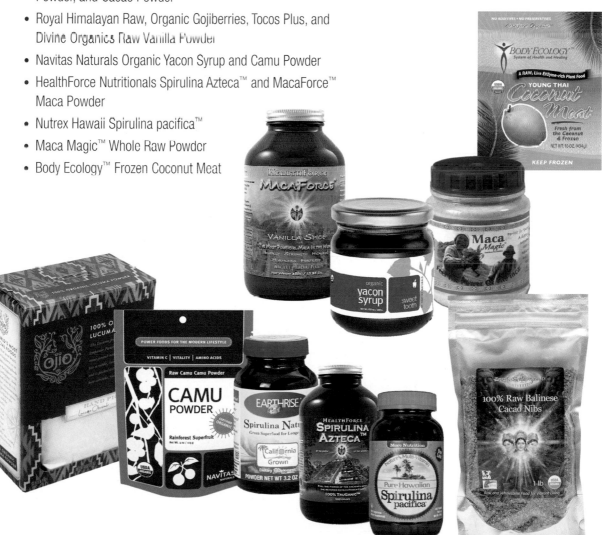

Green, Chai & Black Teas

- Choice® Organic Teas
- Yogi™ Organic Teas
- Guayaki® Organic Yerba Mate
- Mighty Leaf® Organic Teas
- Zhena's Gypsy Tea®

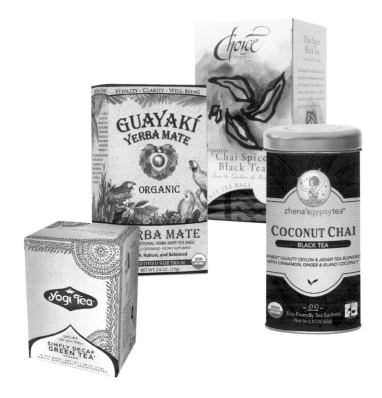

Nut & Seed Butters

- Rejuvenative Foods Raw, Organic Nut and Seed Butters
- Artisana™ Raw, Organic Nut and Seed Butters
- Living Tree Community Foods Alive, Organic Nut and Seed Butters
- Wilderness Family Naturals® Organic, Raw Nut Butters
- Once Again Nut Butters Organic, Raw Butters
- Futters Nut Butters™ Organic, Raw Nut and Seed Butters

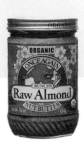

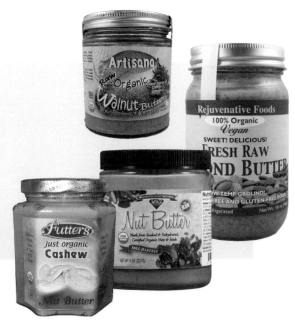

Making Nut & Seed Milks

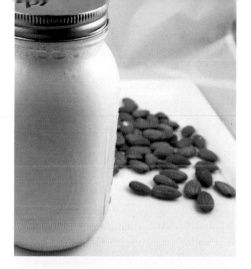

Once you make fresh nut or seed milk, you may find it hard to go back to the pre-made, boxed brands. Freshly made nut milk tastes so authentic and delicious, plus it provides protein, "good" fat, and calcium for strong physical development. Nut and seed milks are a great base for smoothies, soups, dressings, sauces, ice creams, and Naked Bliss shakes. Try a variety of nut and seed milks for their individual properties and unique flavors (see chart on pp. 28 to 30).

Making your own nut and seed milks could be something that you start doing on a regular basis. I make almond milk every three to four days and keep it in my refrigerator. It is an easy, inexpensive, and convenient way to keep fresh, creamy nut milk on hand at all times. For those who are sensitive to tree nuts, the seed-milk options are an excellent substitution, and they are filled with vitamins and minerals. Sure, these may all be purchased in the market and make great, convenient substitutions for dairy milk, but they are not a raw product. And nothing tastes better or provides for a Naked lifestyle better than homemade.

Easy as 1-2-3:

1. Soak the nuts or seeds as directed in the Nuts & Seeds Nutritional Chart (except for varieties that do not need to be soaked).

2. Blend 1 cup of soaked nuts or seeds with 4 cups of purified water.

3. Pour mixture into a nut-milk bag and squeeze to separate the milk from the pulp.

Basic Almond Milk

Makes 3–4 servings
Prep time: 10 minutes

Ingredients

    1 cup whole raw almonds, soaked
    in water 12 hours

    4 cups purified water

Directions

Drain and rinse soaked almonds. Place in a high-speed blender with water and blend until they are completely broken down and a milky color appears. Place nut-milk bag into large pitcher or bowl. Pour nut milk mixture into bag. Close bag and gently squeeze with hands until all liquid is extracted. The remaining pulp may be discarded or frozen in an airtight container. Store nut milk in a glass container in the refrigerator for up to 5 days.

Nuts & Seeds Nutritional Chart

NUT/SEED	1 OUNCE	FIBER	PROTEIN	SOAKING	NUTRITIONAL ASPECTS
Almonds	23 nuts	3g	6g	6–12 hrs	Contain vitamin E, calcium, magnesium, potassium, and zinc. Helpful for bones, brain, heart, lungs, and alkalizing the blood.
Brazil nuts	6–8 nuts	2g	4g	Do not soak	Great source of cysteine, methionine (amino acids), calcium, and selenium. Very good for thyroid.
Cashews	16–18 nuts	1g	4g	1–2 hrs	Loaded with copper, magnesium, tryptophan, and phosphorus. Support the heart, prevent gallstones, and are a good antioxidant source.
Chia seeds	4 tablespoons	11g	4g	5–10 min	Contain omega-3 fatty acids, calcium, potassium, and antioxidants. Increase endurance in athletes.
Hazelnuts	18–20 nuts	3g	4g	6–12 hrs	Rich in calcium and strengthen the teeth and gums. Rich in potassium and vitamin E to aid heart health.

NUT/SEED	1 OUNCE	FIBER	PROTEIN	SOAKING	NUTRITIONAL ASPECTS
Hemp seeds	4 tablespoons	0g	10g	Do not soak	Packed with omega-3 fatty acids. Contain a full complement of amino acids, as building blocks of protein.
Macadamia nuts	10–12 nuts	2g	2g	Do not soak	Loaded with calcium, iron, phosphorus, selenium, and zinc. Rejuvenate the liver, improve anemia, and aid in heart health.
Pecans	20 halves	3g	3g	2–6 hrs	Rich in B-complex vitamins, especially B6. Nourish nervous system. Support pregnant and nursing women.
Pine nuts	140 nuts	1g	4g	1–2 hrs	Loaded with amino acids, B-vitamins, and minerals like copper, iodine, magnesium, and zinc. Help digestion and cardiovascular health.
Pistachios	49 nuts	3g	6g	6–12 hrs	Similar nutritionally to almonds, but are higher in iron and vitamin B1. Support heart, liver, kidneys, and intestines. Great source of protein.

Nuts & Seeds Nutritional Chart, CONTINUED

NUT/SEED	1 OUNCE	FIBER	PROTEIN	SOAKING	NUTRITIONAL ASPECTS
Poppy seeds	4 tablespoons	5g	5g	6–12 hrs	Helpful with anxiety, bronchial problems, coughs, and insomnia.
Pumpkin seeds	150 seeds	0g	5g	6–12 hrs	Rich in omega-3 fatty acids, B-complex vitamins, and calcium. They're great for the heart and improve dry skin and brittle hair.
Sesame seeds	3.5 tablespoons	3g	5g	Do not soak	Contain vitamin E and iron and are high in calcium. Sesame milk is a phenomenal way to prevent osteoporosis.
Sunflower seeds	5 tablespoons	3g	6g	6–12 hrs	Rich in zinc and B-complex vitamins. Support the prostate, heart, intestines, nervous system, and eyes.
Walnuts	14 halves	4g	4g	2–6 hrs	High essential fatty acid content, along with vitamin E, calcium, and potassium. Support heart health.

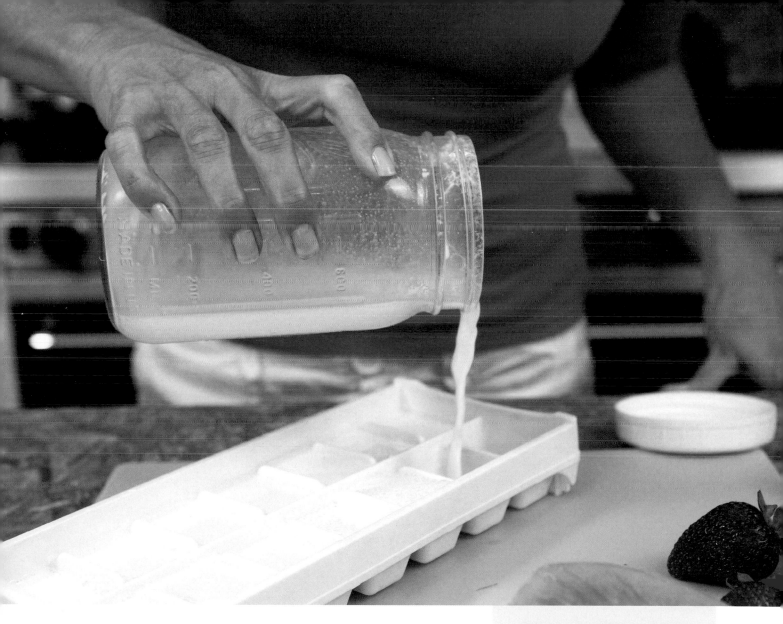

Using Nut Butters Instead of Making Nut Milks

When there is no time to soak and blend your fresh nut milk, or the store-bought carton is empty, you can use 2 tablespoons of raw nut butter with 8 ounces of purified water as your nut-milk base for your milkshake. It may have a slight bit more texture, but it will be yummy.

Make nut-milk ice cubes and use in place of regular ice cubes for a frothy, cool, and extra creamy Blissful shake.

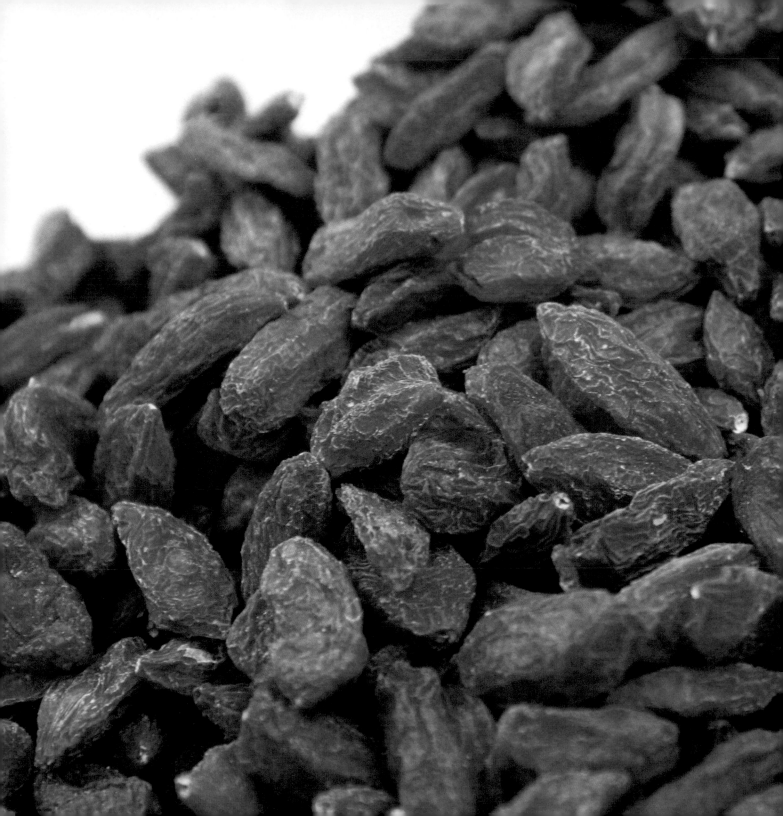

Superfoods

Superfoods are the new paradigm of nutrition. How people saw and valued nutritious food in the past doesn't even touch the benefits that superfoods bring to our health. Superfoods are nutritionally dense, live foods that nourish, energize, cleanse, and heal the body. They are living, raw plant foods, which include most fruits and vegetables, nuts, seeds, seaweeds, sprouts, grasses, fresh herbs, and fermented foods (or cultured foods).

"Superfood" is a new word in nutrition, much like "organic" was more than 10 years ago. Because our culture and this generation have embraced the word "organic" and no longer consider it foreign, markets and grocery stores are being overwhelmed with new organic products every day. To stay within the universal comfort zone of modern eating, however, the requirements for being labeled "organic" have lessened. Consequently, our quality of organic food is no longer optimally nutritional.

The superfoods that I mention here are literally SUPER foods. They are not only indigenous plant foods, freshwater algae, or highly mineralized saps—they are true medicine. Each one of these superfoods has abundant healing properties that can skyrocket your health to a new level.

The next four pages show a short list of easily accessible superfoods that we are fortunate to have in our mainstream markets. If they are not available in local markets, you can order them online. The online world of raw, organic, live, and medicinal foods is booming. You can pretty much "Google" anything and find it at your fingertips. If ever there was a time to get healthy, it is now!

Superfoods offer what no other foods can. How we measure vitamins and minerals is by an obsolete food chart that provides minimal nutritional information. It provides only a small portion of the essential vitamins, minerals, fats, carbohydrates, and so on that matter to our human health. Most people are mineral deficient and nutritionally deprived and are, therefore, lethargic, overweight, or underweight, depending on the mineral depletion. Our culture has an abundance of mysterious inflammations, headaches, pain, skin problems, sleep disorders, and the constant threat of cancer. Superfoods can provide the nourishment to improve vitality, increase life-force energy, and aid and heal the discomfort in our bodies because they provide nutritional elements that even scientists don't understand yet. Superfoods are a silent promise for longevity.

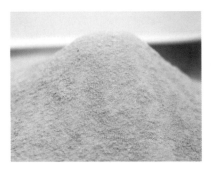

Camu camu: A Brazilian fruit similar to the crabapple, camu camu contains more vitamin C than any other food in the world. It comes from a pristine part of the Amazonian rainforest and is harvested in waterways by canoe. It is a staple in Peru and even China. It was only recently discovered in the U.S. and is being imported as a superfood. It contains 60 times more vitamin C than oranges. It is also very high in iron, potassium, riboflavin, niacin, and phosphorus. Camu camu is a strong antioxidant that exhibits anti-inflammatory activity in the body, and it can protect the liver from damage.

It is sold in a powder form and has a very tart flavor, as you would expect from a vitamin-C source.

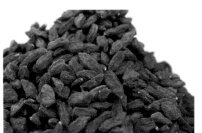

Goji berries: Goji berries have brilliant nutritional value, topping the charts as an all-time favorite because of their anti-aging properties. Goji berries play an important role in detoxifying the body by strengthening the immune system, protecting the liver, and aiding digestion. They enhance the libido by increasing testosterone levels and keeping blood pressure under control.

Goji berries are world famous for their abundant nutrition. They are pretty little red fruits containing 19 amino acids, 21 trace minerals, and an abundance of protein. Loaded with vitamins B and E (which is rarely found in fruits), goji berries contain more antioxidants than any other fruit.

Goji berries may be grown fresh in certain climates or purchased dried, like little red raisins, or in powder form.

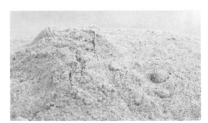

Lucuma: Lucuma was once the "gold of the Incas." It is a Peruvian fruit that's recognized for its high nutritional value as well as delicate flavor. Lucuma powder is an excellent source of carbohydrates, fiber, vitamins, and minerals, including remarkable concentrations of beta-carotene, niacin, and iron. It is a yellowish tropical fruit that has a tasty flavor and aroma that are hard to describe or compare to any other. Some of the comparisons I've seen are butterscotch, maple, pumpkin, or caramel, but none is quite right because the delicate flavor is hard to capture. Its texture, unlike most fruits, is dry, quite starchy, and has a paste-like consistency that melts in your mouth. It is used as a sugar substitute or exotic flavoring.

It is one of the "lost crops" of the Incas and provides super flavor as a superfood.

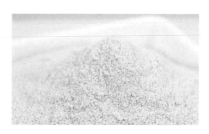

Maca root: Maca, also known as "nature's Viagra™," has eager lovers all over getting some of this sweet, malt-like Peruvian root. Famous for its hormone-balancing and libido-enhancing qualities, Maca has found its home in the marketplace. Maca can also aid with depression, insomnia, fatigue, and acne. It is an adaptogen that can treat symptoms of menopause and sexual dysfunction. (Adaptogens are like shock absorbers for stress, trauma, anxiety, and fatigue.)

Maca has been called the "Peruvian ginseng" because it is legendary for promoting mental and physical vitality. It is known for increasing people's performance, endurance, energy, and stamina in physical activities. It is an excellent superfood for athletes.

Maca is sold as a dried, raw, organic root powder or liquid drops.

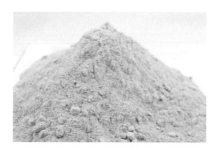

Mesquite pod: Many of the well-known superfoods have a sweetness to them—this is nature letting us know that life is meant to be sweet. Mesquite pod meal is made from the pods of the Peruvian mesquite tree by grinding the seeds and pods to create a sweet, bold-flavored, tasty flour. Mesquite pod may be classified as more of an alternative sweetener than a superfood, but because it is rich in calcium, magnesium, potassium, iron, amino acids, zinc, lysine, omega-3 fatty acids, and soluble fiber and has a 20% to 30% protein content, we are going to label it super.

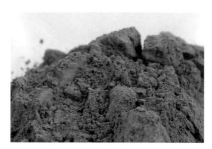

Raw cacao: Raw chocolate has the highest amount of antioxidants of any food in the world. Of course there are other foods that have a similarly high concentration, but they cannot be consumed in quantities enough to have as profound an effect as raw cacao.

It is the superfood that just keeps on giving. Chocolate has long been known for its aphrodisiac, hormone-balancing, and mood-enhancing qualities, but the miracle of the raw version takes chocolate to a whole new level.

Raw cacao is known to benefit a wide range of cardiovascular issues. The antioxidants and abundant amounts of magnesium and other phytochemicals promote general health by balancing blood pressure, lowering high cholesterol, and reversing heart disease. Cacao is the highest whole food source of magnesium, which also happens to be the most deficient mineral in the diet of modern cultures.

Raw cacao is not processed and is available in powder, nib, or whole-bean form.

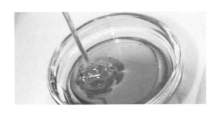

Raw honey/royal jelly: Raw, unprocessed honey is a deeply medicinal food that contains the richest source of live enzymes. The sweet nectar provided by honeybees can increase mental alertness and is known to aid digestion, ulcers, and infection because of its antibiotic effects. Eating cooked honey does not have the same effect, so it is important to eat raw and wild when possible.

Royal jelly is a magical superfood that is not fully understood yet. It is a thick, milky substance secreted by worker bees that is known to regenerate and rejuvenate the body, inhibiting the aging process. Long known as "the fountain of youth and beauty," it contains remarkable amounts of proteins, lipids, vitamins, hormones, enzymes, mineral substances, and specific vital factors that are biocatalysts in cell regeneration within the human body. With as little as ¼ teaspoon of royal jelly a day, you can add years to your life.

(Bee products may cause an allergic reaction in some people, so start with small amounts to test your body.)

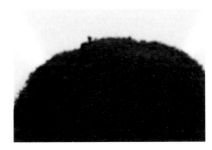

Raw vanilla powder: Vanilla powder is more highly recognized for its rich, aromatic flavor than for being a superfood, but as a magical bean with alluring qualities, it is to be celebrated in the superfoods list.

Vanilla is one of the oldest and most expensive spices. It is a bean that comes from the exquisite blooms of the vanilla orchid. The bean is cured by the sun and then ground at a low temperature, keeping the fragrant powder potent and luscious. Vanilla serves as an antioxidant and has nonspecific healing properties that can enhance your mood and libido. It calms the mind and the nerves, which in and of itself has tremendous healing power.

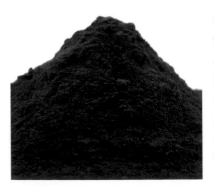

Spirulina: Spirulina is the most nutrient-dense food on the planet. It is a freshwater, single-cell, blue-green algae that is a complete protein source. Just 1 tablespoon provides 10 grams of protein and all 8 essential amino acids. It has the highest concentration of beta-carotene of any food and contains other immune-supporting elements found in no other food. It is a powerhouse for balancing brain chemistry, the liver, and nervous system, along with purifying the blood and strengthening joints. When we eat green superfoods that are nutritionally balanced, such as spirulina, this translates into balance throughout the body.

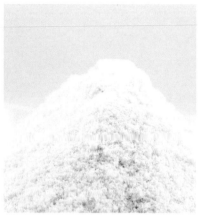

Tocotrienols powder:

Tocotrienols are a balanced, whole food made from rice bran that provides stable nutrients and a full protein complement. Tocotrienols are members of the vitamin E family. There are more than 100 known antioxidants in tocotrienols, plus naturally occurring selenium, CoQ10, alpha lipoic acid, flavonoids, glutathione peroxidase, essential fatty acids, vitamins, minerals, and enzymes that help protect the body from the formation of free radicals and degenerative disease. It is mild tasting, which makes it highly usable because it won't change the taste of anything to which you add it. It is easily digestible as well as soothing and nutritive for even the most distressed digestive systems. It is an excellent way to boost your nutritional protocols.

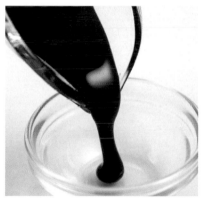

Yacon root:

Yacon is a low-glycemic, natural sweetener that contains inulin, which is a naturally occurring probiotic found in plants that serves as a fertilizer for good bacteria in the lower intestines. It contains a special kind of fructose, called fructo-oligosaccharides, which cannot be absorbed by the body. It provides great benefits as a probiotic food, feeding the friendly bacteria, boosting the immune system, and helping digestion. It contains a superfood level of antioxidants, placing it prominently on the superfood list.

Yacon is related to the Jerusalem artichoke and sunflower and has a rich molasses flavor. Yacon syrup can be used like agave, honey, or maple syrup.

Is Bacteria Really 'Friendly'?

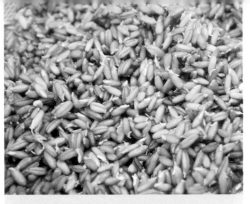

There is a lot of talk about probiotics, lactobacillus, acidophilus, and other "friendly" bacteria, and for good reason. Good bacteria builds a healthy colon and a healthy colon helps eliminate toxins. Probiotics strengthen the immune system and aid in overall digestion.

Because rejuvelac is a fermented culture, you should observe, smell, and taste it periodically to become accustomed to the changes that occur over time.

Rejuvelac is a probiotic drink that is full of friendly bacteria. It is a fermented liquid that is used to improve digestion and health, increase energy, and aid in an overall sense of well being. It is a live, organic, non-dairy source of 45 billion acidophilus enzymes that help your body assimilate nutrients and eliminate toxins. It is loaded with B vitamins, vitamins E and K, a variety of proteins, carbohydrates, phosphates, and amylases (rich digestive enzymes).

Rejuvelac serves many functions in the body:

- Protects against bad bacteria, yeast growth, and infections
- Produces and absorbs vitamins, enzymes, and oxygen
- Improves skin health
- Corrects digestive dysfunction

It is a raw food prepared by sprouting grains and then soaking the grains in room-temperature water for a couple of days. The liquid can be consumed as a digestive aid or used as a starter for other fermented foods such as nut and seed cheeses.

Rejuvelac tastes like a tangy, sugar-free lemonade. It has a slightly yeasty, fermented smell, but the flavor is tart and non-offensive.

I blend it with the dairy-free ice creams to get a yogurt-like flavor. I use it in many of my Naked Bliss recipes, so prepare a batch today. It will last several weeks in your refrigerator.

Rejuvelac

Rejuvelac is best prepared using whole wheat, rye, or quinoa grains. You can combine them or use just one. I prefer the wheat and rye mixture.

Makes 2 litres • Prep time: 2–5 days

Ingredients

  1 cup wheat berries, rye berries, or quinoa

  1 quart filtered water for soaking

  8–10 cups purified water

Directions

First soak the grains for 1 day in 1 quart of filtered water.

Drain the water and pour the berries into a fine mesh strainer, nut-milk bag, or sprouting bag. Place over a bowl for drainage.

Rinse berries with cool water up to 7 times a day for up to 3 days until tails form. They are now sprouted.

Place sprouted berries in a gallon container and add 8 to 10 cups of purified water. Cover with gauze or cheesecloth for protection, but do not cover with a lid. Let sit for 1 to 3 days (fermentation will occur faster in a warm climate) as the water becomes murky and a slight foam develops on top.

Strain through cheesecloth or nut-milk bag.

Will last 2 to 3 weeks in glass jars in refrigerator.

Rejuvelac should have a pleasant, yeasty smell with a lemony flavor.

Drink a glass of rejuvelac each day to improve bowel flora.

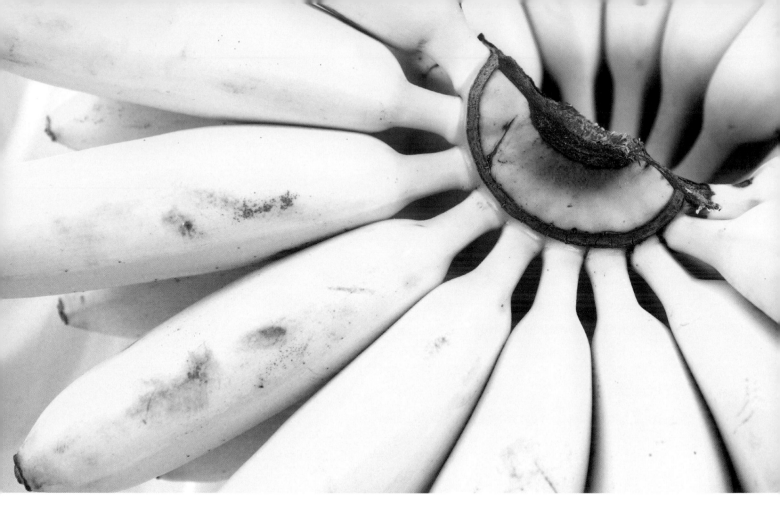

Gone Bananas

I'll bet you didn't know that bananas don't grow on trees. I didn't, either. They actually grow on compacted, water-filled leaf stalks that grow up to 25 feet high. They are the world's largest herb.

Bananas are one of those things that add a delicate sweetness to your life and fill you with satisfaction. They are America's number-one favorite fruit and are the most largely consumed fruit in the country since winning the hearts of the people over apples in the 1900s. Bananas contain considerable amounts of vitamin B6, vitamin C, and potassium. They are also great for replenishing your electrolytes when you live an active lifestyle. There are more than 1,200 varieties of bananas worldwide, but we see only a few of these beauties in our local marketplaces.

Cavendish banana: This widespread banana makes up more than 95% of the bananas sold in the U.S. They are the official "dessert banana," with a mild taste and mushy texture when fully ripened. They ripen naturally and are at their peak when the peel is yellow with a few dark-brown specks.

Baby banana (bananitos): These are smaller and sweeter than the Cavendish banana, which makes for a fun little "Scooby snack" when hunger strikes. When ripe, they have bright-yellow skin and cream-colored flesh.

Manzano (apple banana): These are my personal favorite as they are small and have nutty, pearl-like seeds inside. They are said to have a strawberry-apple flavor. I don't taste that subtlety, I just like them. They are less starchy and sweet than the classic Cavendish and seem to digest with greater ease. These fruits must be very ripe to reach full sweetness; their skin should look deep brown with dark streaks. Brown bananas are not very popular to grocery shoppers, but if you don't let them ripen to full potential you will be disappointed. It's worth the wait.

Red banana: This is one of the most delicious bananas in the marketplace. If you are lucky to find them on your grocer's shelf, buy them up. The red banana has a sweet taste and a creamy texture. The ripeness of a red banana can be tough to gauge; look for dark-magenta ones with streaks of umber. Their flesh bruises easily, so handle with care.

Burro: This is a chunky banana, stubbier and fatter than the Cavendish. This banana is grown in Mexico and is usually found in Latin American markets. It is good to ripen it a long while to enjoy the full extent of its sweet-and-sour taste, which I've always thought of as a cross between a lemon custard pie and banana cream pie.

Plantain: Plantain bananas may look like other bananas, but the resemblance ends there. Plantains are very starchy and not very sweet. They are a kind of banana that is usually cooked. With a few exceptions, these rarely reach the eat-raw sweetness of varieties like Cavendish. In many cultures, the degree of ripeness determines how a particular variety is eaten—it may be cooked if green and eaten raw when ripe.

Whenever you feel overwhelmed or confused, simplify!

· ·

**Banana plants are the largest plants on Earth without a woody stem.
They are actually giant herbs of the same family as lilies, orchids, and palms.**

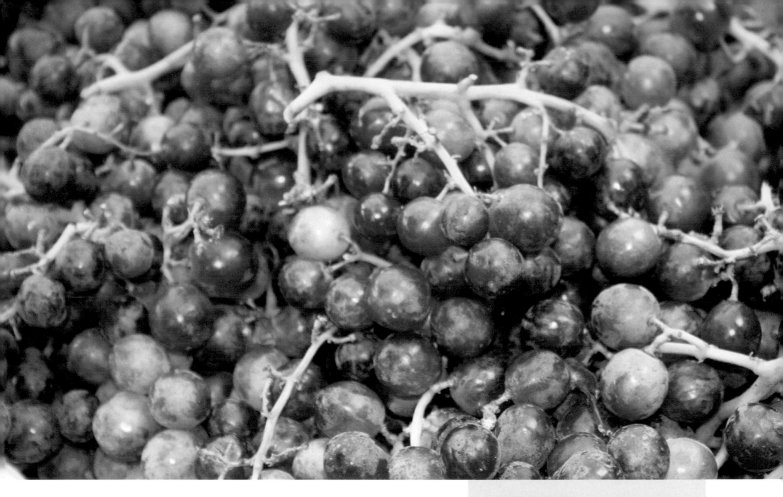

Fruits With Seeds

Ugly is the new pretty. Smitten with beauty, our culture has driven the evolution of foods to be altered to please the eye as well as the palate. What nature has provided as perfect has been changed to be ultra-perfect. No seeds, no fuzz, and no bitter tastes. Unfortunately, those changes are only skin deep. Genetically engineered or hybridized foods have become devoid of proper minerals that the once-wild version had. Be proactive—pick the fruits that have seeds, especially when choosing watermelon, grapes, and citrus fruits. Even bananas should have a little black, walnut-like seed inside. Find that ugly duckling in the sea of pretty produce and know that it will provide you with a little extra something for your own beautiful self.

> Biblical verse Genesis 1:29
> *~New 2007 Translation~*
>
> **Then God said, "Look! I have given you every seed-bearing plant throughout the Earth and all the fruit trees for your food."**

Fresh & Fruity

Fresh, seasonal fruit added to a Blissful shake makes for an impressive and stunning meal. The body derives so much energy from fresh fruit, and fruit digests quickly, keeping the metabolism rolling. I love fruit shakes when I want something light, refreshing, and uplifting.

Enjoy experimenting with your favorite seasonal fruits.

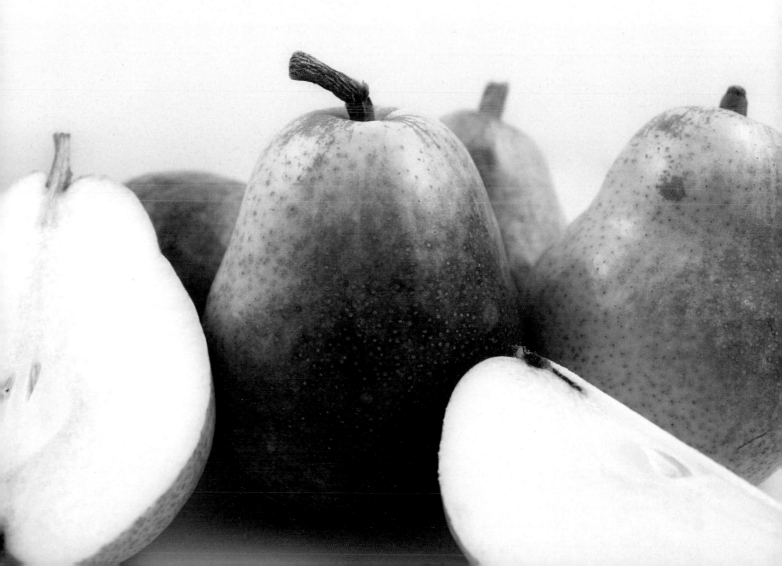

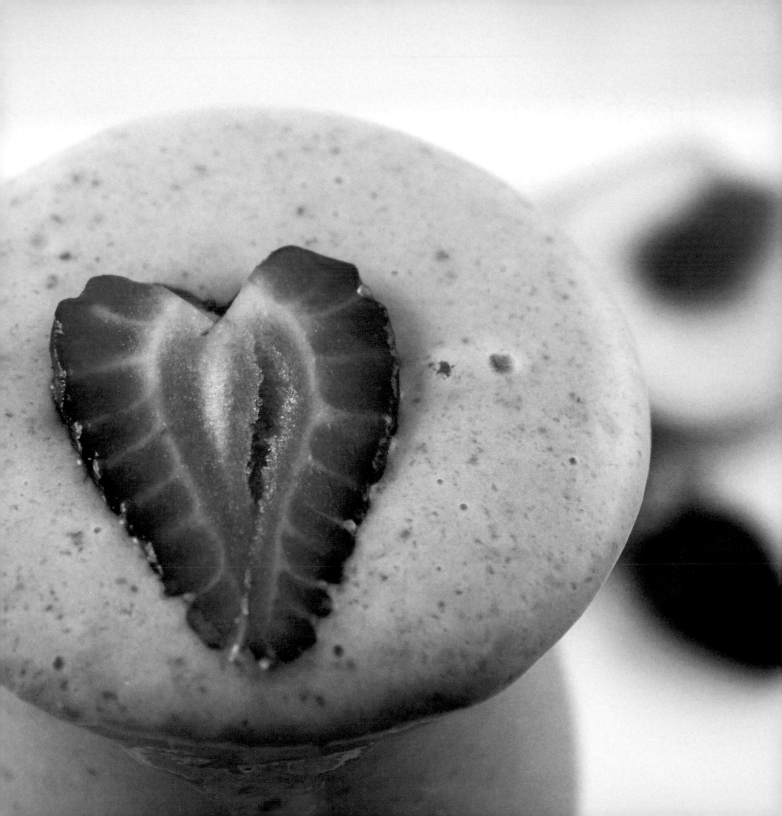

Strawberry Peach Daiquiri

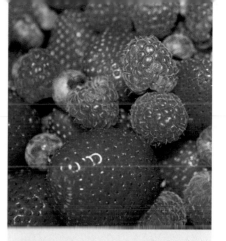

Makes 1–2 servings • Prep time: Less than 5 minutes

Every time I make this, someone says, "This is my favorite taste combination." There is something about the delicious taste of fresh fruit that is undeniable. Just like a daiquiri made with tangy fruit and sweet whipped cream, this shake has that delicate balance between tart and creamy. I don't know about you, but this is one of my favorite taste combinations, too.

Ingredients

    1 cup Coconut Bliss Vanilla Island

    ½ cup almond milk (or nut or seed milk of choice)

    1 pint fresh strawberries

    1 cup peaches

Directions

Place almond milk and fresh fruit in blender to liquefy, then add your Bliss and blend.

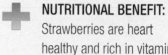

FUN FACT: Strawberries remove dental plaque and whiten teeth without damaging enamel.

NUTRITIONAL BENEFIT: Strawberries are heart healthy and rich in vitamin C and folate.

HOW TO SELECT: Choose organic strawberries with a rich, red color.

Just Plum Good

Makes 1–2 servings • Prep time: Less than 5 minutes

What else would one name something this good? It's just plum good!

It tastes a bit like a plum tart with melted ice cream oozing over the top. Use any type of plum you like, and remember to keep the skin on.

Ingredients

1 cup Coconut Bliss Vanilla Island

½ cup almond milk (or nut or seed milk of choice)

1 cup diced black plums

½ teaspoon cinnamon

Directions

Blend all ingredients on high until smooth and creamy.

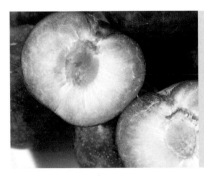

 FUN FACT: Plum trees are grown on every continent except Antarctica.

 NUTRITIONAL BENEFIT: Plums contain high amounts of vitamin C, and they stimulate the bowels.

 HOW TO SELECT: Avoid plums that are discolored, leaky, too soft, or appear shriveled.

Nutrients in black plums are easily digested and absorbed by human bodies.

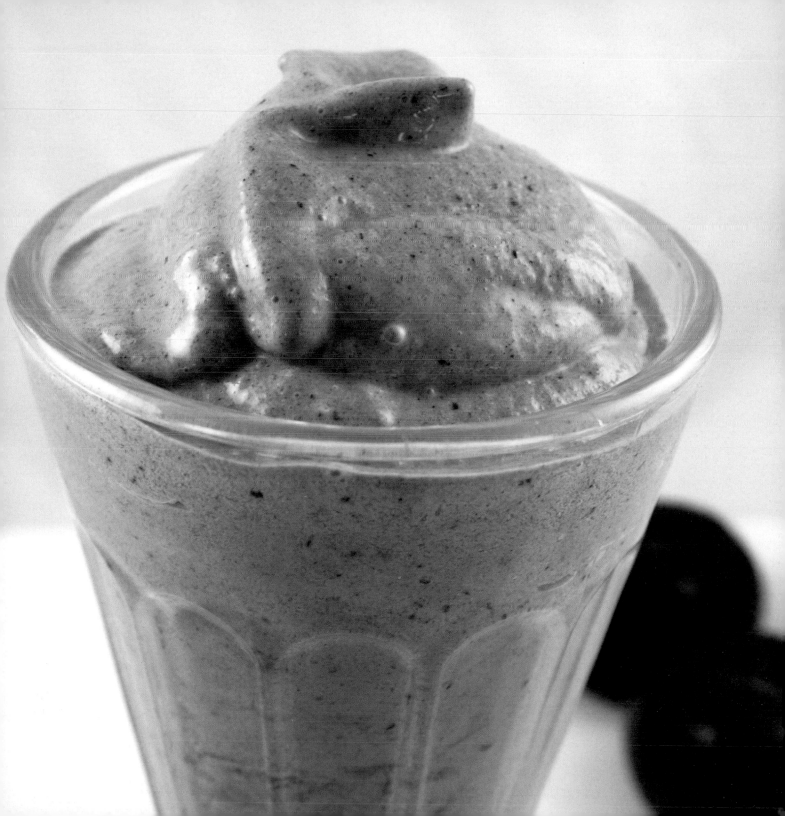

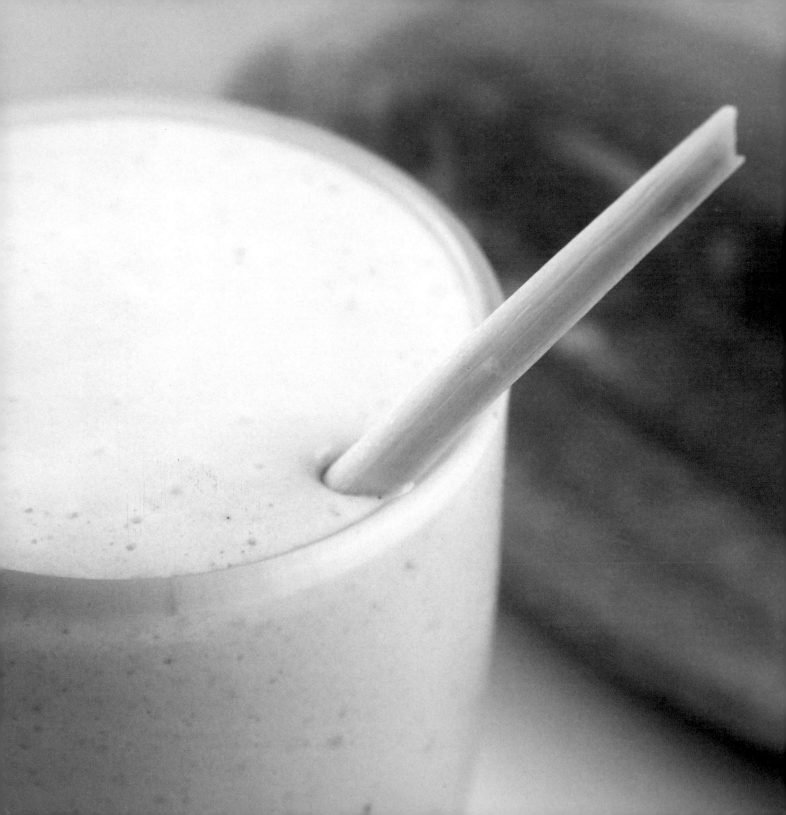

Papaya Lemongrass

Makes 1–2 servings • Prep time: 5–10 minutes

Papaya is such a wonderful tropical fruit, plus it contains the active enzyme papain that helps you digest protein. It's super delicious when mixed with a tart fruit, such as citrus. But when you add grated lemongrass to it, you get a unique flavor and the most amazing tonic for the tummy. With or without your Bliss, this is a keeper. I suggest adding the ice cubes to this shake because the papaya can make it a bit thick and the ice lightens the drink.

Ingredients

1 cup Coconut Bliss Vanilla Island

½ cup almond milk (or nut or seed milk of choice)

1 cup fresh papaya

1 teaspoon grated lemongrass

1 cup ice cubes (optional)

Directions

Blend all ingredients on high until smooth and creamy.

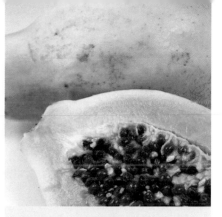

FUN FACT: Meat tenderizer is composed mainly of an enzyme extract from the papaya, called papain.

NUTRITIONAL BENEFIT: Papaya aids digestion and acts as a diuretic and laxative.

HOW TO SELECT: Look for skin that is turning from green to yellow. Parts of the papaya may look bruised; this is normal.

You can blend the papaya seeds in with the papaya. They add a peppery taste and have unique anti-parasitical properties.

Lemongrass, also known as citronella, can relieve stress and insomnia.

Cran-Apple

Makes 1–2 servings • Prep time: Less than 5 minutes (or up to 20 if you're pressing your apples fresh, and well worth it)

This is one of the best combinations ever made, in my opinion. The tartness of fresh or frozen cranberries with the sweetness of fresh-pressed apple juice makes for a creamy and delicious shake. Cranberries are only in season for a short time, so you will want to stock up and freeze them for the year to follow.

Ingredients

1½ cups Coconut Bliss Vanilla Island

1 cup fresh-pressed apple juice

½ cup cranberries

Directions

Blend all ingredients on high until smooth and creamy.

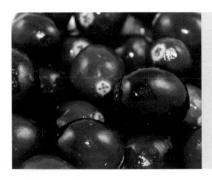

 FUN FACT: Cranberries were once called "bounceberries" because they bounce when ripe.

 NUTRITIONAL BENEFIT: Cranberry juice can help prevent urinary tract infections.

 HOW TO SELECT: Choose deep-red berries with firm skin.

Buy cranberries in season and freeze them in an airtight container to use for the rest of the year.

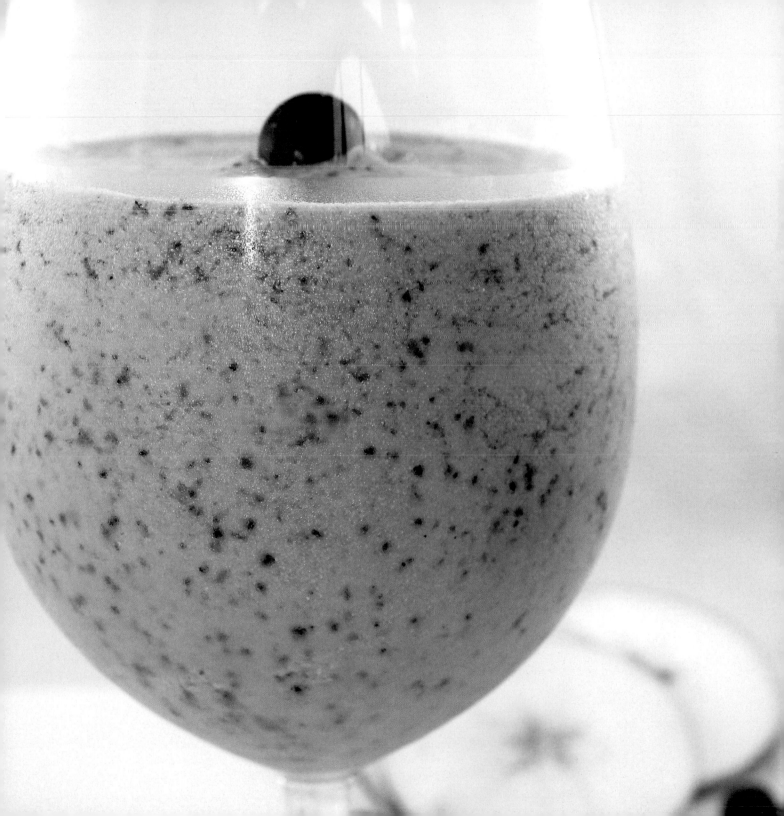

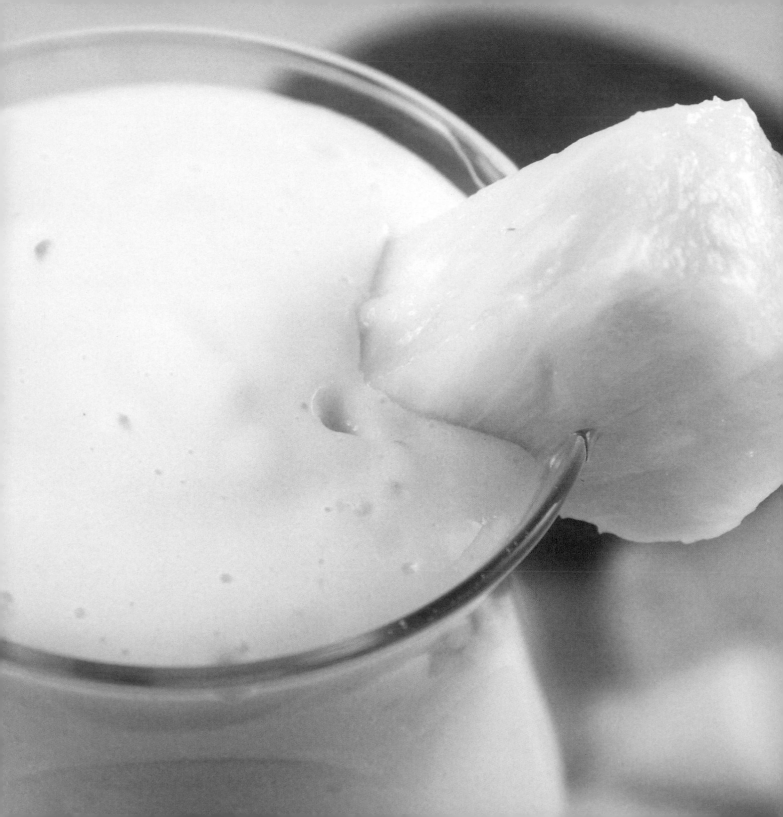

Tropical Bliss

Makes 1–2 servings • Prep time: 5–10 minutes (or more if you're juicing your oranges fresh)

Creating the taste of the tropics is easy when you mix coconut and pineapple together, but when you add a bit of fresh orange juice and mango, you make this tropical drink a dream come true. If you are not squeezing your own oranges, make sure that you buy unpasteurized juice from your local market so that you get all the benefits of fresh juice.

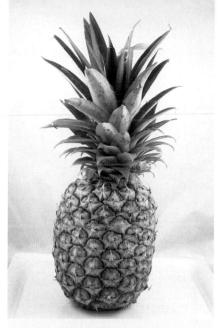

Ingredients

1 cup Coconut Bliss Pineapple Coconut

½ cup freshly squeezed orange juice

1 mango, diced

1 cup pineapple

1 cup ice cubes (optional)

Directions

Place orange juice and fresh fruit in blender to liquefy, then add your Bliss and blend. Blend in ice cubes if you like it frothy and light.

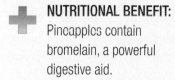

FUN FACT: Fresh pineapple can to be used as an enzyme wash for your face.

NUTRITIONAL BENEFIT: Pineapples contain bromelain, a powerful digestive aid.

HOW TO SELECT: Choose pineapples by smelling the underside for sweetness.

If you like a thick, frothy shake and you use fresh fruit, you may need to add ice cubes.
Instead of regular ice cubes, try substituting nut-milk ice cubes.

Blackberry Bliss

Makes 1–2 servings • Prep time: Less than 5 minutes

Blackberries are deep, dark, and mysterious. They only come out for a short time each year and yield the most incredible juicy and plump fruits. With their unique structure adding to the nutritional content, blackberries provide more fiber than most other fruits.

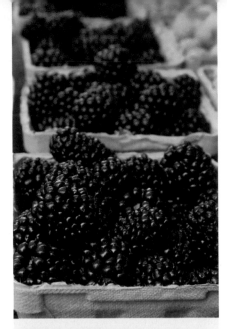

Ingredients

    1 cup Coconut Bliss Vanilla Island

    1 cup blackberries

    ½ cup almond milk (or nut or seed milk of choice)

    ½ cup rejuvelac (see p. 39)

    ½ frozen banana

Directions

Blend all ingredients on high until smooth and creamy.

FUN FACT: Wild blackberries have thorns.

NUTRITIONAL BENEFIT: Blackberries are an effective treatment for nausea.

HOW TO SELECT: Look for berries that are firm, yet fully ripe.

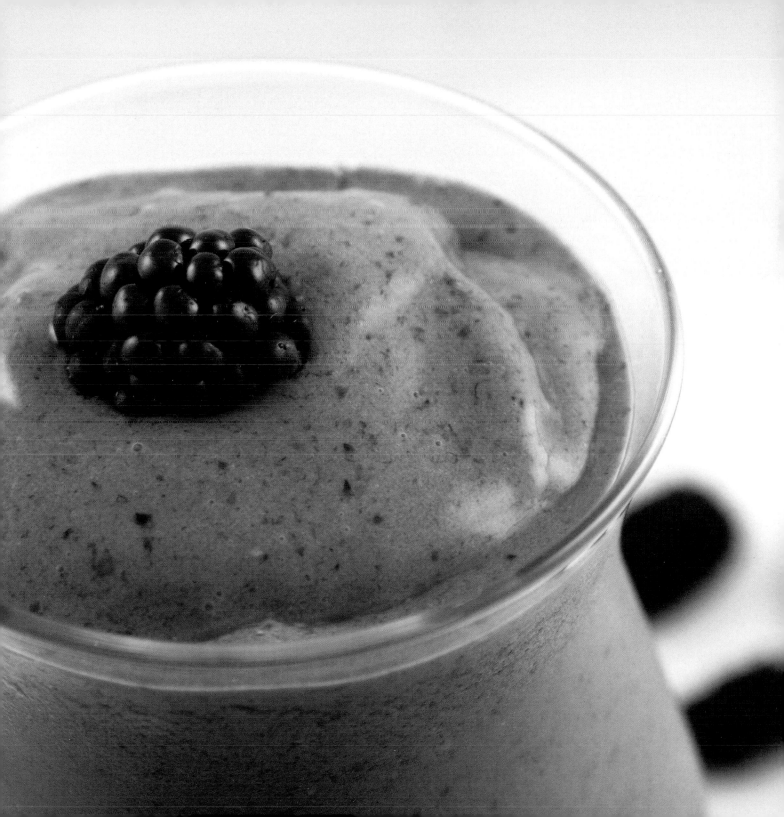

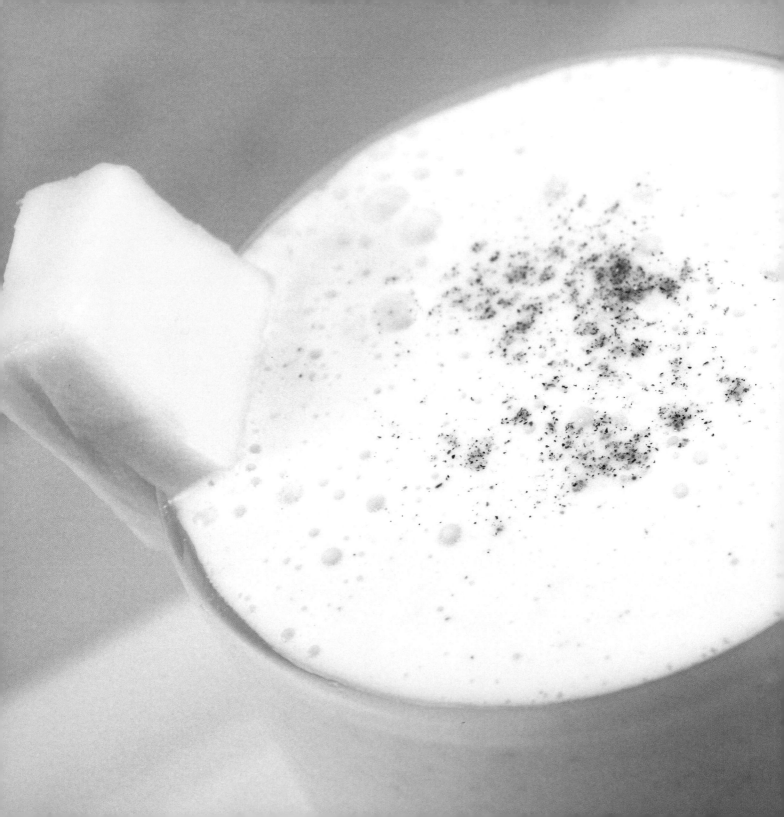

Mango Lassi

Makes 1–2 servings • Prep time: Less than 5 minutes

This Indian-inspired drink will help you achieve deep spiritual enlightenment. And if that doesn't occur then bless it first. It tastes so good you will start worshipping it as a favorite amongst your repertoire. It is tangy mango creaminess at its finest.

Ingredients

1 cup Coconut Bliss Vanilla Island

½ cup almond milk (or nut or seed milk of choice)

½ cup rejuvelac (see p. 39)

1 cup fresh mango, diced

⅛ teaspoon ground cardamom pod

Directions

Blend all ingredients on high until smooth and creamy.

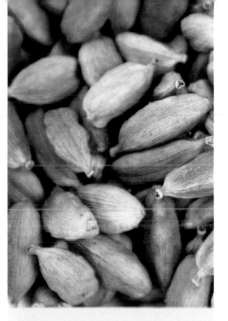

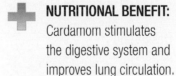

FUN FACT: In *The Canterbury Tales*, cardamom is called "the spice of paradise."

NUTRITIONAL BENEFIT: Cardamom stimulates the digestive system and improves lung circulation.

HOW TO SELECT: When possible, choose organic cardamom in the pod or seed.

Mango has antiviral, antiseptic, and anti-parasitical properties.

Mango Raspberry Bliss

Makes 1–2 servings • Prep time: Less than 5 minutes

Really, you could put any fruit with raspberries, or add mango to just about anything, and it would taste good. But when you combine these two highly charged, super-antioxidant fruits together, the flavors burst and your energy soars. Be creative and mix and match fruits of your choice.

Ingredients

    1 cup Coconut Bliss Vanilla Island

    ½ cup almond milk (or nut or seed milk of choice)

    1 cup fresh mango, diced

    1 cup raspberries

Directions

Place almond milk and fruit in blender to liquefy, then add your Bliss and blend.

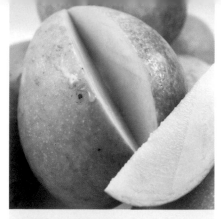

FUN FACT: Mangos are a symbol of love, and some believe that the mango tree can grant wishes.

NUTRITIONAL BENEFIT: Mangos are high in vitamin C when green. Their vitamin A content increases as they ripen.

HOW TO SELECT: Pick a fragrant mango that is plump and heavy for its size.

Raspberries are considered an aphrodisiac because of their hormone-stimulating properties.

Remember—when you use frozen fruits, you may need to add more liquid or reduce the amount of fruit for each shake.

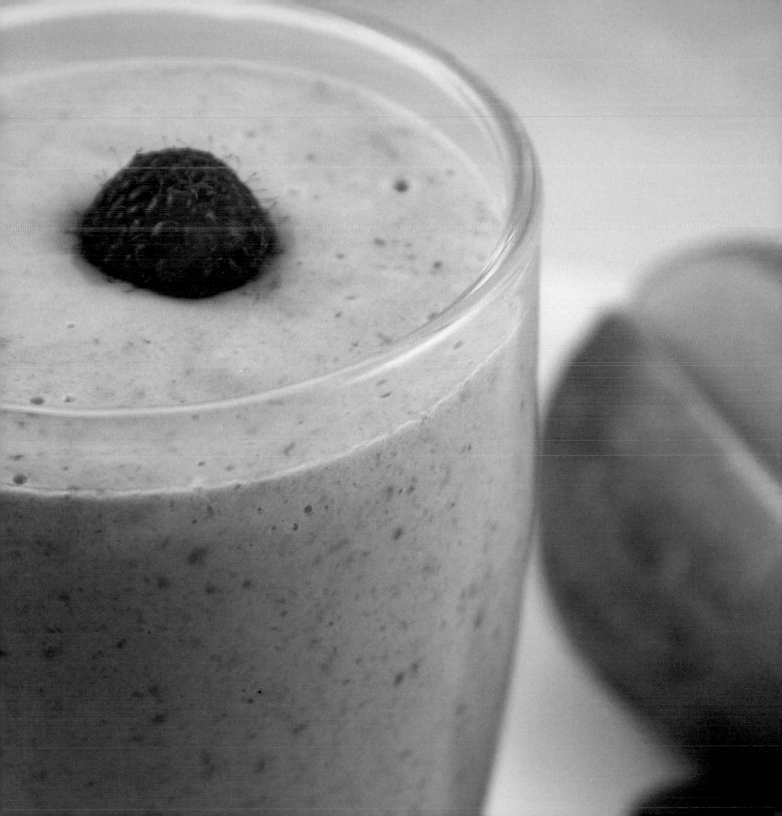

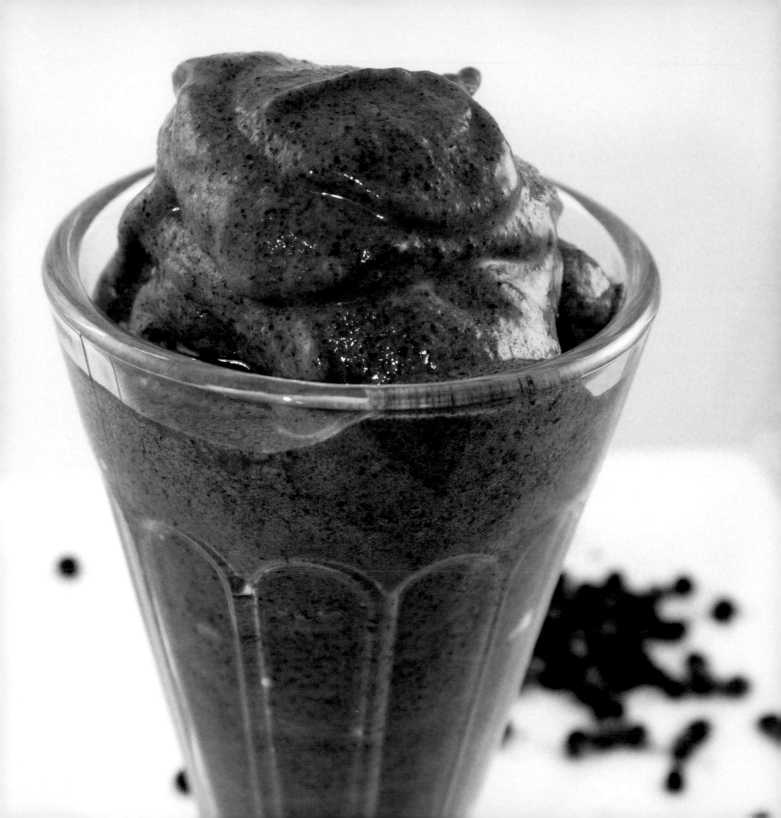

Blueberry Bliss

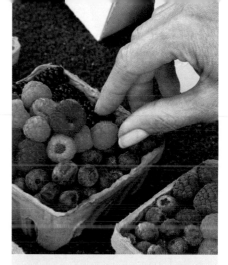

Makes 1–2 servings • Prep time: Less than 5 minutes

Nothing beats blueberries for an antioxidant boost, and the flavor is oh so sweet. By adding a probiotic drink to this smoothie, you also get tartness and a boost of friendly flora for your digestion.

Ingredients

1 cup Coconut Bliss Vanilla Island

1 cup blueberries

1 cup rejuvelac (see p. 39)

2 Medjool dates, pitted

Directions

Blend all ingredients on high until smooth and creamy.

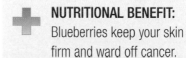

FUN FACT: Blueberry skins were once mixed with milk and used as paint for Shaker wood houses.

NUTRITIONAL BENEFIT: Blueberries keep your skin firm and ward off cancer.

HOW TO SELECT: Look for fresh blueberries that are firm, dry, plump, and smooth-skinned with a deep purple-blue to blue-black color.

Take the worry out of your life and open yourself to new sensations of pleasure.

To Juice or Not to Juice?

That is the question.

Pure pressed juices that are sold in the marketplace are flash pasteurized. This means that they are quickly heated to about 160°F (70°C) and then immediately cooled, all within a matter of seconds. This process destroys microorganisms and denatures enzymes, minimizing chemical and physical change. Flash pasteurization allows for a longer shelf life in the refrigerator and ultimately establishes a convenience.

Fresh-squeezed juices in some produce sections or farmers' markets have not been heated and, therefore, are a good option to keep around the home. They may only last 3 to 5 days in the refrigerator before they begin to ferment, but they give you the active enzymes that aid good health. This is a "live" food.

Juicing for life, from raw organic produce that you drink on the spot, is the ultimate for your health. Whenever possible, go with this method and enjoy the sensation of fresh, live produce entering your body.

It is perfectly fine to fall into the convenience of market juices. It is essential that a Naked lifestyle be user friendly and available at your fingertips. Your overall health and wellness will thrive over time with the small changes of "getting Naked."

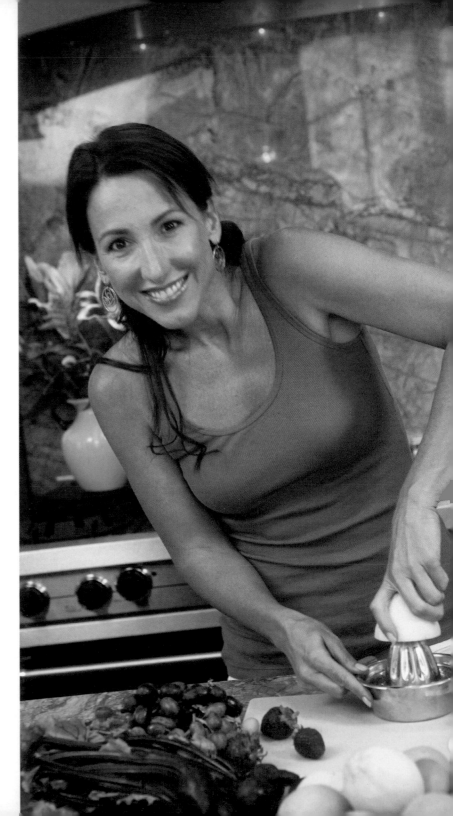

Veggie Dreams

I can't help but think of the nursery rhyme, "Mary, Mary, quite contrary, how does your garden grow? With silver bells, and cockle shells, and pretty maids all in a row." It's such a blissful thought of a beautiful garden and lovely and lively produce blossoming on the earth. When did vegetables become taboo for many in their nutritional health? There is nothing more alkalizing and satisfying than fresh greens. If we can make fresh greens taste like dessert, perhaps more people will eat them. This section is created with poetry and rhymes in mind—to bring back the Bliss in our "veggie dreams."

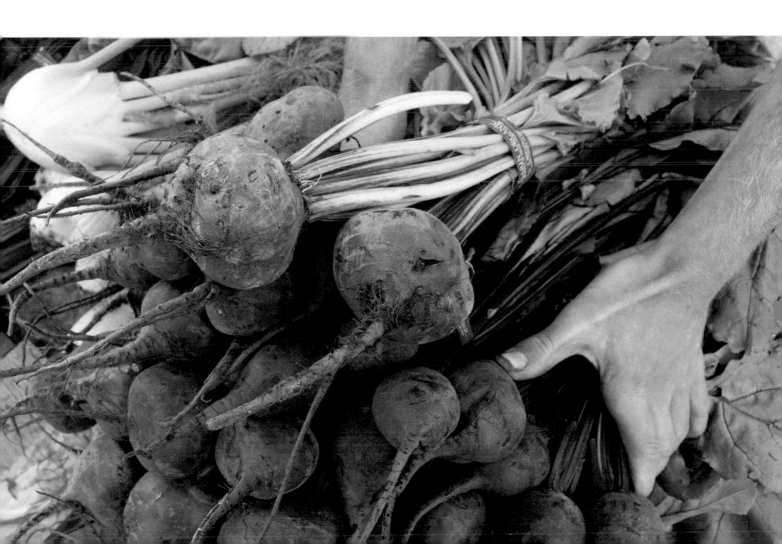

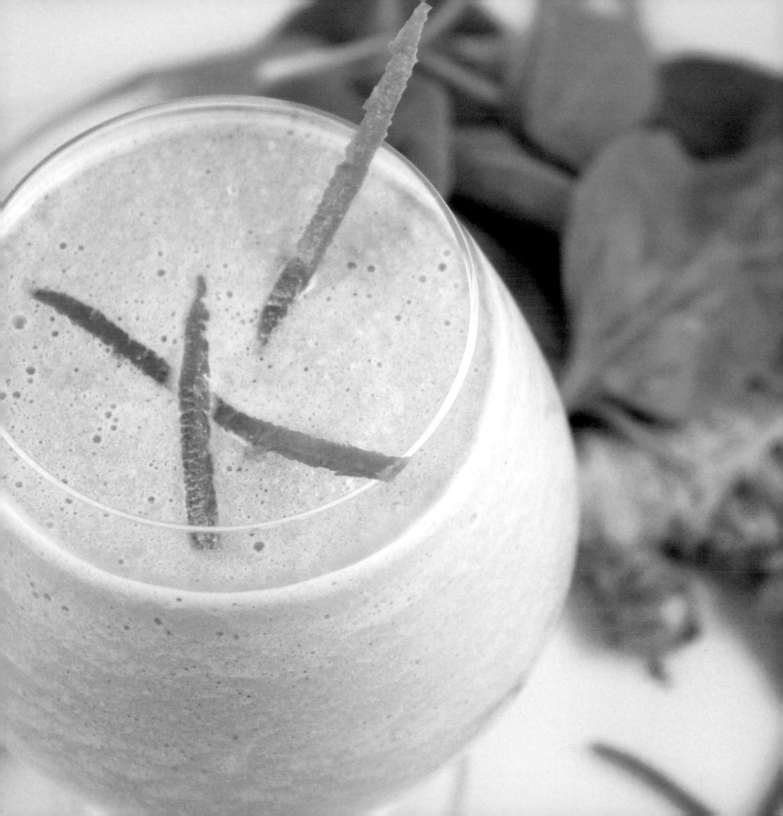

Garden Bliss

Makes 1–2 servings • Prep time: 5 minutes (or up to 20 if you're juicing your carrots fresh)

I plucked some veggies fresh from my garden and made this shake. It was a bit more effort to make my carrot juice fresh, but well worth it. If you find Garden Bliss to be particularly amazing, as I do, then you may want to save time by substituting freshly juiced carrot juice from the market. And feel free to add more ginger—it will get the blood moving and warm you up.

Ingredients

1½ cups Coconut Bliss Vanilla Island

1 cup fresh carrot juice

1 cup fresh spinach

½ teaspoon freshly grated ginger

½ cup ice cubes

Directions
Blend all ingredients on high until smooth and creamy.

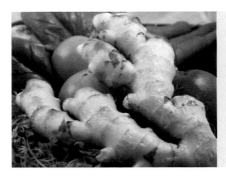

FUN FACT: Ginger is the oldest plant used for medicinal purposes.

NUTRITIONAL BENEFIT: Ginger has been shown to reduce nausea.

HOW TO SELECT: Look for plump ginger with thin, beige skin.

The part of the ginger root that is closest to the center has the most intense flavor.

Lettuce C

Makes 1–2 servings • Prep time: 5 minutes (or longer if you're juicing your oranges fresh)

Take a look at the super-C ingredients listed (oranges and kiwi) and you will know how I got the name for this amazingly energizing and delicious shake. The butter lettuce adds hydration nutrients and a light and refreshing taste to this recipe. If you want an even bigger boost of vitamin C, try adding camu camu (a vitamin C–rich fruit from the Amazonian rainforest) or fresh berries.

Ingredients

1½ cups Coconut Bliss Vanilla Island

1 cup freshly squeezed orange juice

2 kiwifruits, peeled

1 cup butter lettuce

2 Medjool dates, pitted

1 teaspoon spirulina (optional)

Ice cubes (optional)

Directions

Place juice, kiwi, lettuce, and dates in blender and liquefy. Add your Bliss, boost, and ice and blend for a perfect shake.

 FUN FACT: The kiwifruit is actually a berry discovered 700 years ago in China.

 NUTRITIONAL BENEFIT: Kiwifruit benefits respiratory health and reduces coughs and runny noses.

HOW TO SELECT: Choose kiwifruit with no bruises, soft spots, or wrinkles.

Living lettuce should be stored in its original container and rinsed well immediately before using.

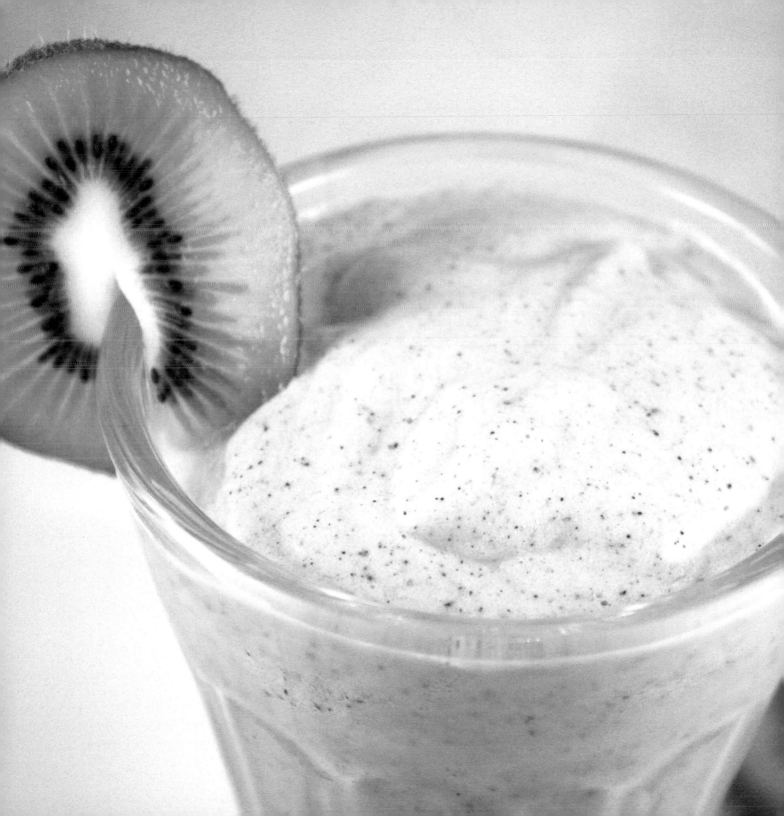

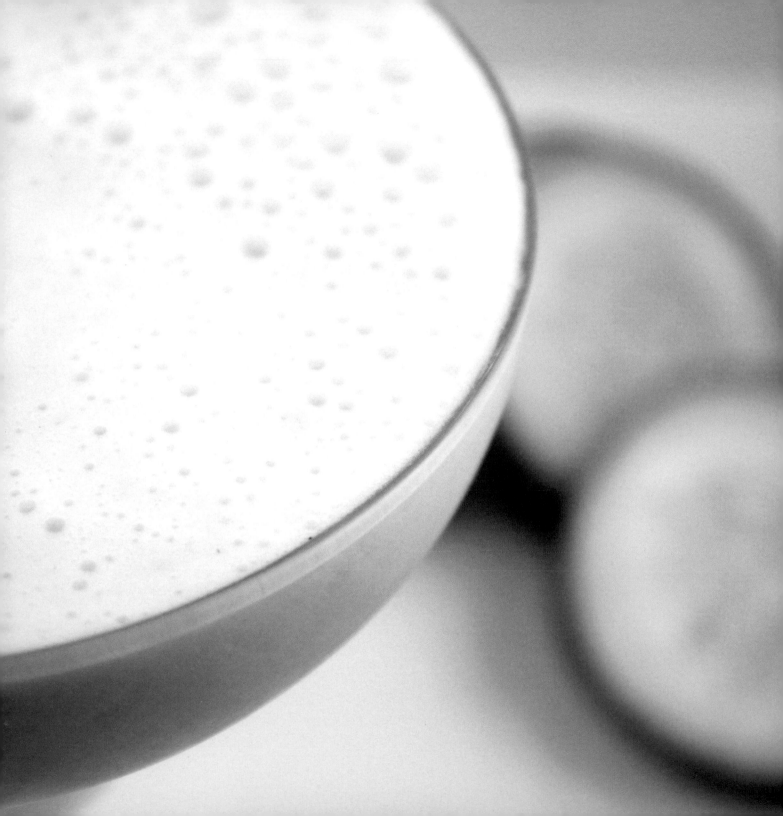

Cool as a Cucumber

Makes 1–2 servings • Prep time: Less than 5 minutes

This is like a creamy cucumber margarita, or at least that is what I tell myself. It's light and refreshing, plus the cucumber hydrates you while the lemon alkalizes your body.

Ingredients

1 cup Coconut Bliss Vanilla Island

1 Bartlett or d'Anjou pear, cored and sliced

1 small cucumber (about 1 cup diced)

1½ tablespoons lemon juice or juice of 1 lemon

Ice cubes (optional)

Directions

Blend all ingredients on high until smooth and creamy.

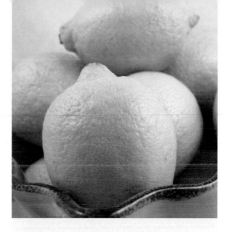

FUN FACT: Lemons at room temperature yield more juice.

NUTRITIONAL BENEFIT: Lemons are high in vitamin C and fiber and help stimulate the liver.

HOW TO SELECT: Look for lemons that are heavy for their size and have a fine-textured peel.

For beautiful, healthy skin, eat cucumbers—they are rich in silica.

"Botanically speaking, tomatoes are the fruit of a vine, just as are cucumbers, squashes, beans, and peas." ~*Horace Gray, an avid horticulturalist who helped create the Boston Public Garden in the 1840s*

Popeye's Cream Dream

Makes 1–2 servings • Prep time: 5 minutes (or longer if you're juicing your oranges fresh)

If Popeye had a blender, he would have dreamt up this creamy concoction. It's so ridiculously outstanding, it truly is a green dream come true.

Ingredients

1½ cups Coconut Bliss Vanilla Island

1 cup freshly squeezed orange juice

2 cups fresh spinach

½ teaspoon vanilla powder

½ teaspoon maca powder

2 Medjool dates, pitted

Directions

Blend all ingredients on high until smooth and creamy.

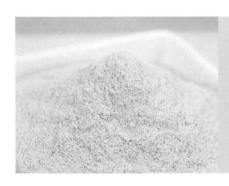

 FUN FACT: Peruvian warriors ate maca root before battle to increase their strength and endurance.

 NUTRITIONAL BENEFIT: Maca nourishes the adrenal glands, heals chronic panic and anxiety disorders, and balances hormones.

 HOW TO SELECT: Know the source of your maca as it can mold easily, even before purchase.

Your body absorbs the iron in spinach poorly unless you eat it with vitamin C.

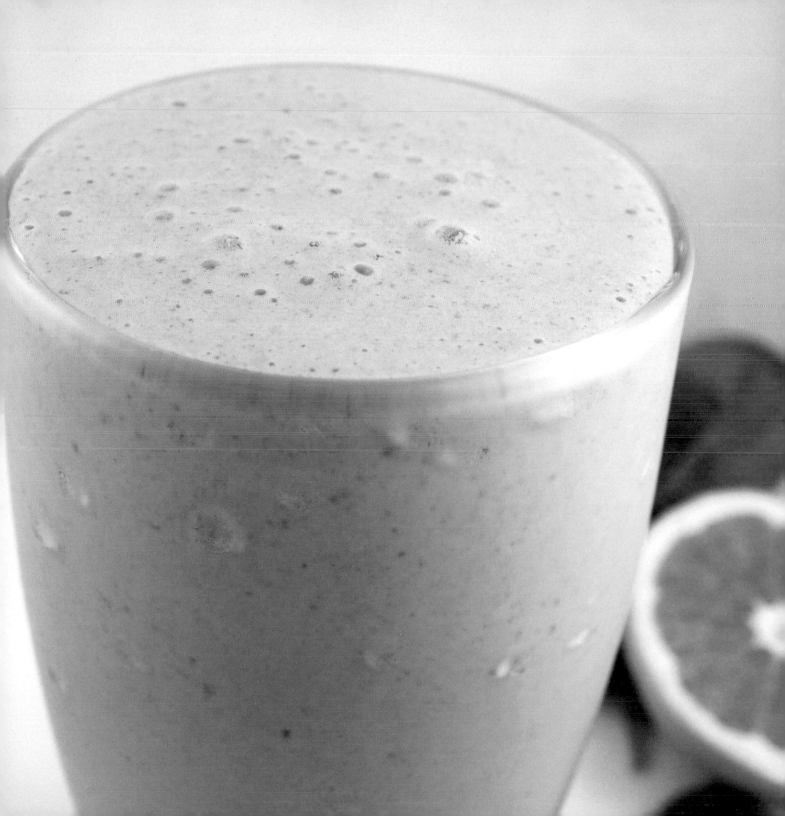

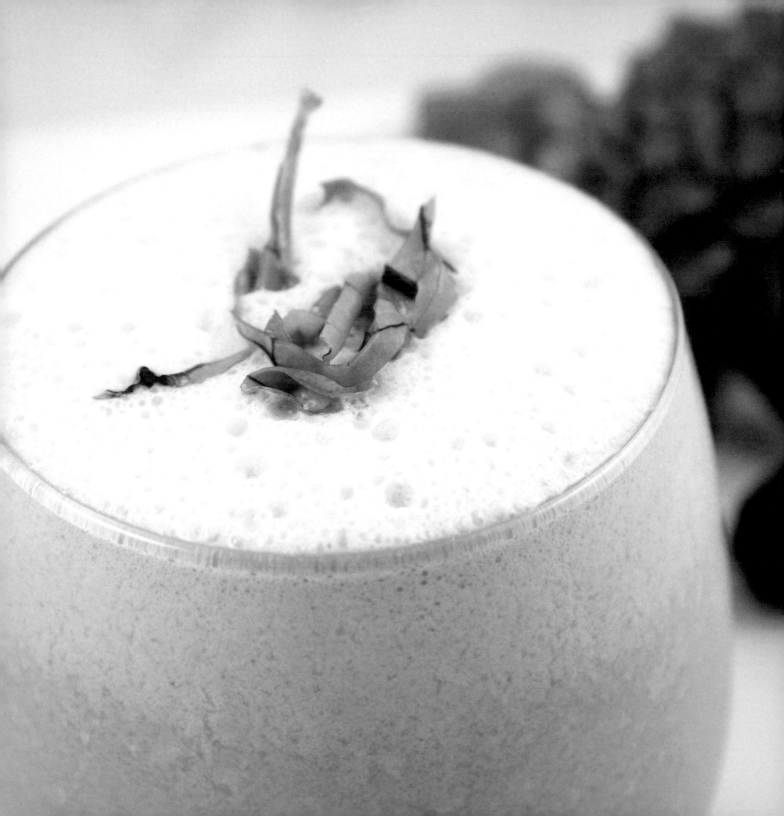

Rainbow Cream

Makes 1–2 servings • Prep time: Less than 5 minutes

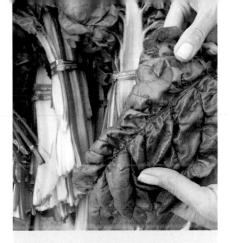

This is rainbow chard at its finest. Chard is so good for you, and there are many ways to incorporate it into a smoothie. The combination in this shake will have you shaking with delight. You won't believe how good chard tastes in a dessert drink.

Ingredients

1 cup Coconut Bliss Vanilla Island

½ cup almond milk (or nut or seed milk of choice)

½ cup rejuvelac (see p. 39)

2 large rainbow chard leaves

2 Medjool dates, pitted

Directions
Blend all ingredients on high until smooth and creamy.

FUN FACT: Chard was discovered by a Swiss gardener who first thought they were special beet greens.

NUTRITIONAL BENEFIT: Chard is an exceptional source of iron, vitamin A, and potassium.

HOW TO SELECT: Choose firm and vibrant leaves.

Be mindful, there is no shortcut to health and happiness.

Kale Colada

Makes 1–2 servings • Prep time: Less than 5 minutes

This is the very first Coconut Bliss recipe I ever created, and it is the very thing that inspired me to continue making Blissful shakes. I held tastings at various health food markets, and the public went crazy for this version of a Hawaiian classic. So, if you like piña coladas …

Ingredients

½ cup Coconut Bliss Vanilla Island

1½ cups coconut water

1 cup pineapple chunks

1 cup Lacinato (also called Dinosaur) kale (about 4 leaves)

Ice cubes (optional)

Directions

Blend on high for 60 seconds and serve immediately.

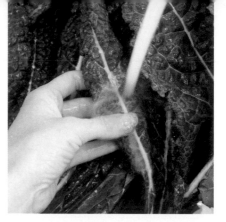

FUN FACT: Once called "poor people food," kale can be grown in even the poorest soil conditions.

NUTRITIONAL BENEFIT: Kale eases lung congestion, benefits the stomach, and is a healer of the liver and immune system.

HOW TO SELECT: When choosing kale, look for a deep green color. Avoid any limp or yellow leaves.

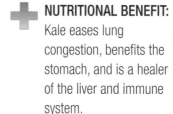

Coconut water is the greatest natural source of electrolytes.

Kale is a power-packed superfood and natural detoxifier.

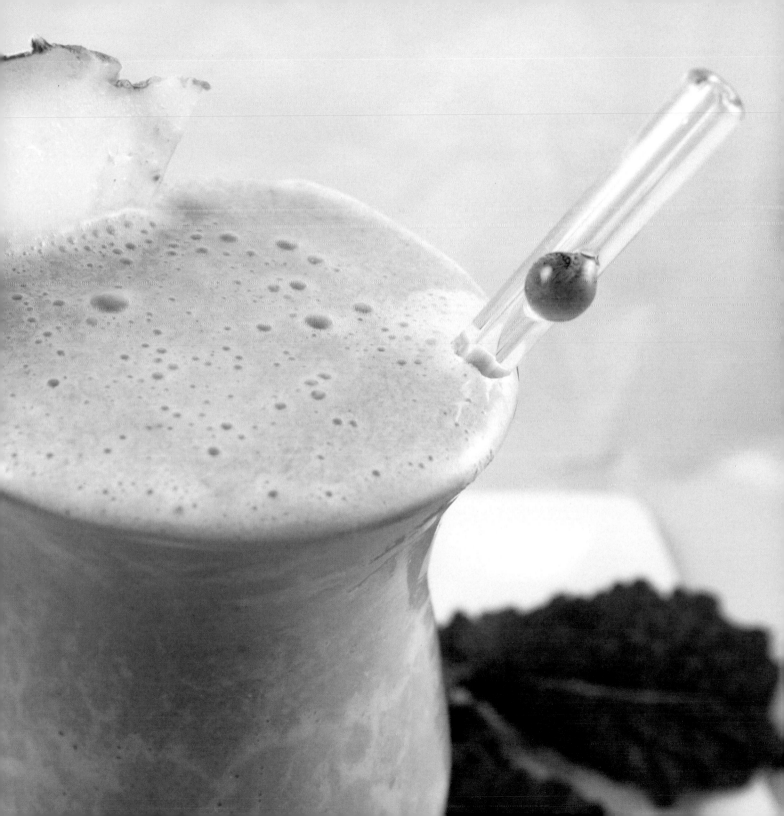

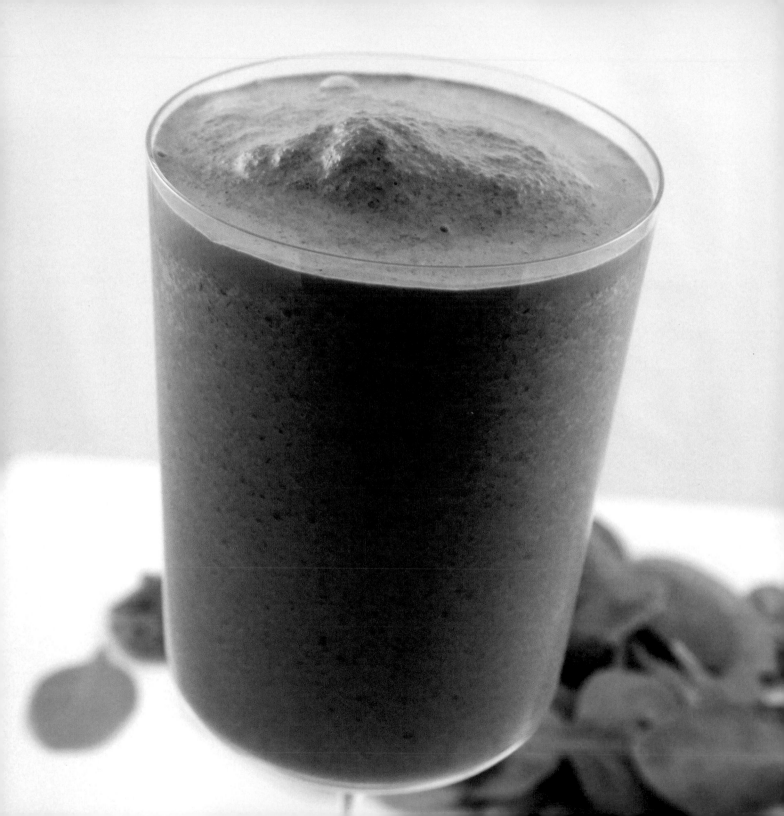

Beet It

Makes 1–2 servings • Prep time: Less than 5 minutes (or up to 20 if you're juicing your beets fresh)

I love beets, as do most people with a sweet tooth. They are a high-sugar vegetable that not only sweetens but colors food to make it visually stunning. Adding the beet greens to this shake along with the spinach will boost the nutrients even higher. If it were me, I would double up on the greens, but make it as you like it!

Ingredients

1½ cups Coconut Bliss Vanilla Island

1 cup beet juice

1 cup fresh spinach (and a few beet greens, if you like)

Ice cubes (optional)

Directions

Blend all ingredients on high until smooth and creamy.

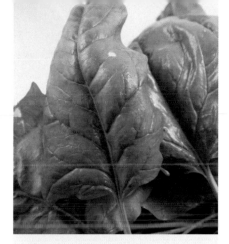

FUN FACT: Spinach belongs to the goosefoot family along with beets and chard.

NUTRITIONAL BENEFIT: Spinach contains more protein than any other vegetable.

HOW TO SELECT: Choose spinach with tender, green leaves. When purchasing spinach, buy organic.

Spinach is an easy plant to grow and has the most nutrition when used fresh.
It loses much of its nutritional value when stored for too long.

Lettuce Sea U Smile

Makes 1–2 servings • Prep time: 5 minutes (or longer if juicing your oranges fresh)

This will really make you smile. It's crisp and light with the right amount of vitamins, protein, and probiotics to make it so good for you. This shake will not only hydrate you, it may become the shake you rely on for a healthy tummy pick me up that satisfies your sweet tooth as well.

Ingredients

1½ cups Coconut Bliss Vanilla Island

½ cup orange juice

½ cup rejuvelac (see p. 39)

2 cups chopped romaine lettuce (about 6 large leaves)

1 teaspoon spirulina

Directions
Blend all ingredients on high until smooth and creamy.

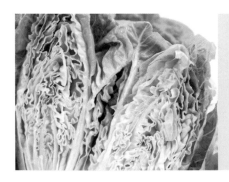

 FUN FACT: Lettuce juice was used as a medicine by many ancient herbalists.

 NUTRITIONAL BENEFIT: The dark-green romaine leaves contain lutein, which supports eyesight.

 HOW TO SELECT: Choose lettuce that has been stored in a misted cooler at the grocery. Avoid heads with wilted leaves.

There are 10 grams of protein in one tablespoon of spirulina. So don't be shy, add more if you like.

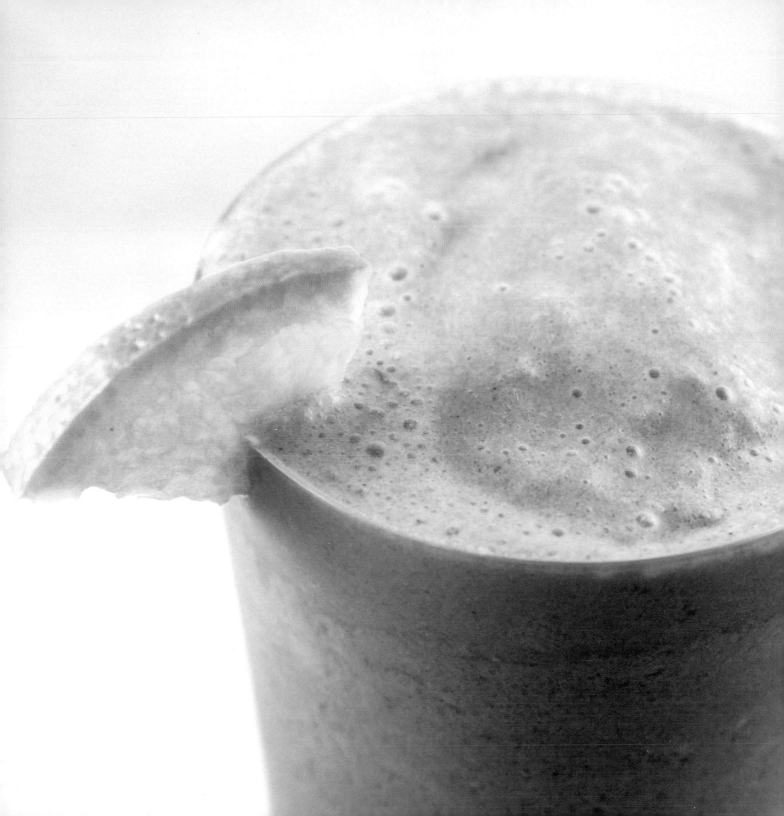

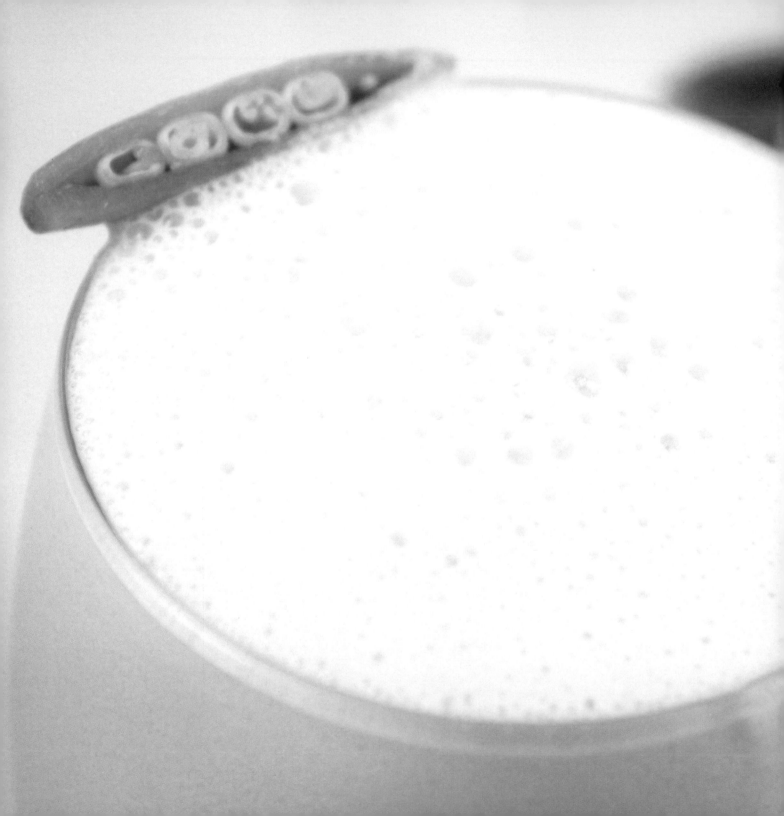

Sweet Pea

Makes 1–2 servings • Prep time: Less than 5 minutes (or longer if pressing your apples fresh)

I love the delicate flavors of sweet pea greens and sugar snap peas. All spring peas for that matter are super nutrient dense and delicious. I like the greens right when they flower; adding them to this shake gives you a burst of blossoming life-force energy.

Ingredients
- 1 cup Coconut Bliss Vanilla Island
- 1 cup freshly pressed apple juice
- 1 cup sugar snap peas (and/or sweet pea greens, when in season)

Directions
Place apple juice with the peas in blender to liquefy, then add your Bliss and blend to perfect creaminess.

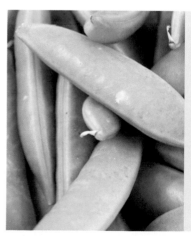

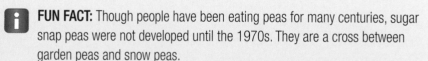

FUN FACT: Though people have been eating peas for many centuries, sugar snap peas were not developed until the 1970s. They are a cross between garden peas and snow peas.

NUTRITIONAL BENEFIT: Green peas help you feel more energetic by providing nutrients that support the energy-producing systems of the body.

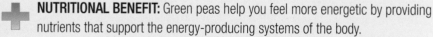

HOW TO SELECT: Make sure the snap peas are fresh by snapping one open. They should be firm and plump. Sweet-pea greens should be used when freshly picked. They tend to quickly toughen and lose their sweetness.

The simpler things are, the easier it is to live.

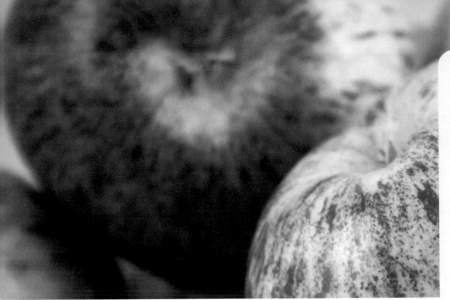

An Apple a Day Keeps the Doctor Away!

There is so much truth to this old proverb, which was meant as good advice for healthful eating.

The truth is that apples digest quicker than any other fruit; they move through your digestive tract in only 20 minutes. As they go, they clean and purify your system with pectin, a soluble fiber that helps increase intestinal viscosity and aid in digestive disorders. Even before modern science verified apples' healthful qualities, people knew that they could heal ailments. When scientists discovered that apples are composed of more than 300 compounds that flood the body with nutrients, the proverb became a modern-day nutritional mantra.

There are more than 7,500 apple varieties grown worldwide. More than 2,500 varieties are grown in the United States alone, and only 100 are grown commercially. The most common varieties are listed to the right.

- **Empire:** This is a McIntosh apple crossed with a Red Delicious for a unique taste.
- **Fuji:** Fujis are very firm and unusually sweet. The skin has red and green stripes.
- **Gala:** These are sweet and very flavorful with orange-striped skin and yellow flesh.
- **Ginger Gold:** These are outstanding early season apples, fresh from the orchard. They are sweet, juicy, and firm.
- **Golden Delicious:** These light-yellow apples are sweet and mellow.
- **Jonagold:** This is a blend of tart Jonathon and sweet Golden Delicious. It's one of the world's favorites.
- **Jonathon:** These apples are juicy and moderately tart.
- **McIntosh:** This bright-red apple is juicy and slightly tart.
- **Mutsu (Crispin):** This large, yellow apple is a cross between a Golden Delicious and an Indo. It's sweet, juicy, and firm with crisp, white flesh.
- **Red Delicious:** The ever-popular Red Delicious is sweet and juicy with dark-red skin.
- **Rome:** The Rome apple is firm and slightly tart. It keeps well and is great for baking.
- **Stayman:** These are firm with a rich, mildly tart flavor. They're a great, all-purpose apple.
- **York:** Known for their distinctive, lop-sided shape, Yorks are crisp, firm, and tart. They keep well and tend to sweeten in storage.

Nostalgic Bliss

So many times I want to eat something that has beautiful memories attached to it, and so many times my digestion reminds me that not all memories are blissful. Nostalgic Bliss is about classic flavors that remind us of wonderful times spent with loved ones: sitting by the fire, huddling with family, laughing, celebrating, and feeling the utmost joy of being alive. There is never a good reason to miss out on the memories of good old traditional flavors.

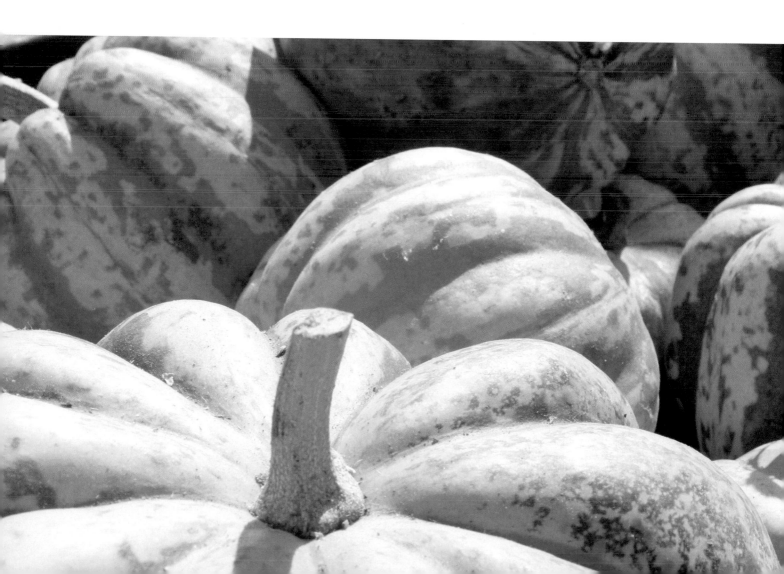

Apple Pie & Ice Cream

Makes 1–2 servings • Prep time: Less than 5 minutes

It doesn't get more nostalgic than this. Quick—what moment crosses your mind when you think of fresh apple pie and ice cream? I know for me it is having Grandma visit and spending the day in the kitchen with her. The magic of the senses and emotions we attach to food comes through in the most blissful way with this nurturing shake. Enjoy some for me.

Ingredients

1 cup Coconut Bliss Vanilla Island

1 apple, cored and peeled (or leave the peel on the apple for optimal nutritional value)

½ cup rejuvelac (see p. 39)

½ teaspoon cinnamon

½ teaspoon pure vanilla powder

Pinch of nutmeg

Directions
Blend all ingredients on high until smooth and creamy.

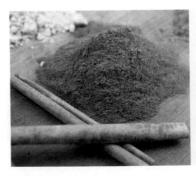

FUN FACT: Cinnamon is a main ingredient in the "bubble gum" flavor.

NUTRITIONAL BENEFIT: Cinnamon is a supreme digestive tonic.

HOW TO SELECT: If possible, select organic cinnamon sticks and grind them just prior to use.

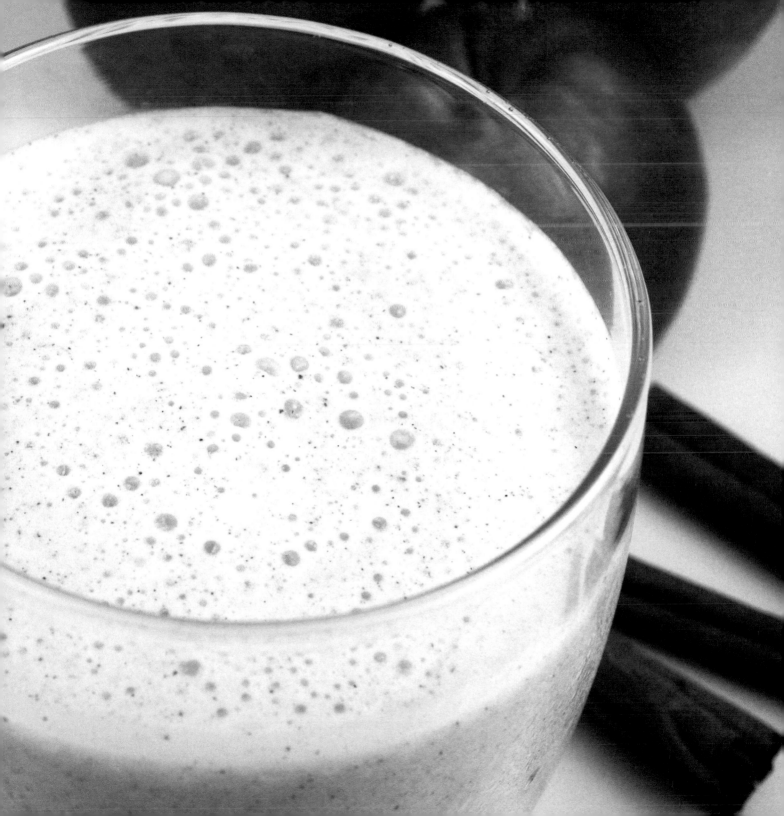

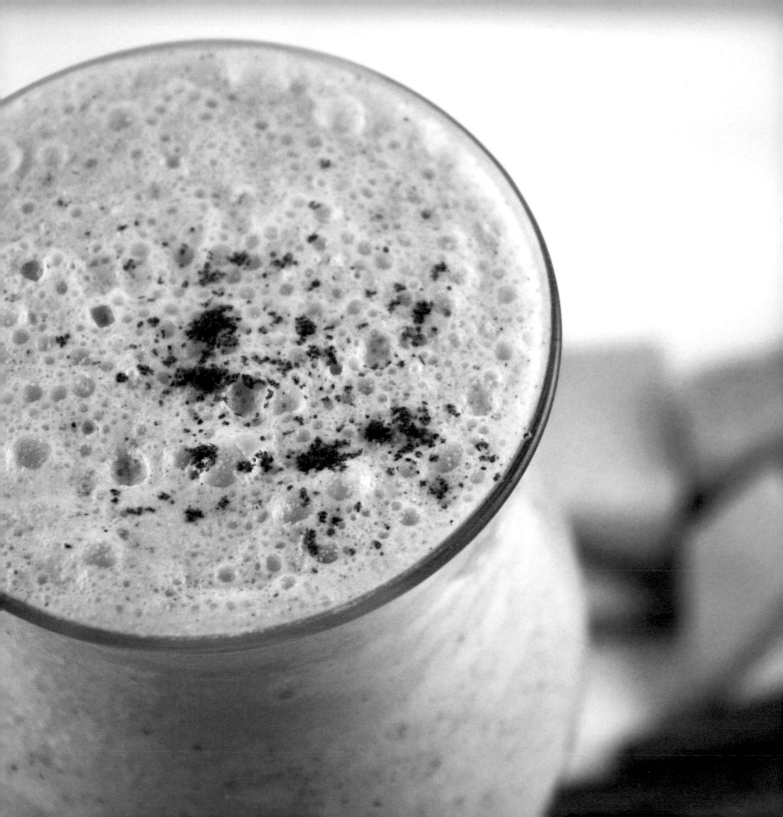

Pumpkin Pie Spice

Makes 1–2 servings • Prep time: 5 minutes (or longer if juicing your carrots fresh)

As soon as October hits, I think pumpkins. I think jack-o'-lanterns and pumpkin pie. If you like pumpkin pie, you will love this shake. Although it is made with carrot juice, it has just the right amount of spices that make you tingle with the comforting flavor of pumpkin pie.

Ingredients

1½ cups Coconut Bliss Vanilla Island

1 cup fresh carrot juice

½ teaspoon cinnamon

⅛ teaspoon nutmeg

⅛ teaspoon ground cloves

Ice cubes (optional)

Directions

Blend all ingredients on high until smooth and creamy.

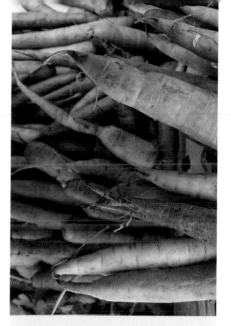

FUN FACT: Young, fresh carrot tops can be juiced or used in fresh salads.

NUTRITIONAL BENEFIT: Carrots are an excellent source of vitamin A.

HOW TO SELECT: Choose carrots that are smooth, firm, and bright in color.

Spices have more disease-fighting antioxidants than most fruits and vegetables.

Caramel Apple

Makes 1–2 servings • Prep time: 5 minutes (or longer if pressing your apples fresh)

This creamy and tart shake topped with a caramel swirl is so reminiscent of those fall flavors we love so much. What a wonderful idea for a holiday party for some added fun. Multiply the caramel sauce recipe for other uses—it will keep for a while.

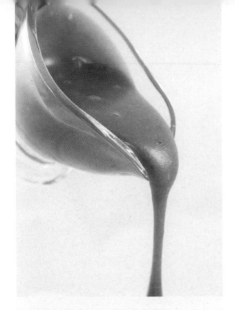

Ingredients

1½ cups Coconut Bliss Vanilla Island

1 cup fresh-pressed apple juice

1 tablespoon lucuma powder

1 tablespoon maple syrup

Directions

Blend all ingredients on high until smooth and creamy.

Caramel Sauce

Ingredients

1 teaspoon lucuma powder

1 teaspoon maple syrup

Directions

Mix together in a small bowl or ramekin until a caramel paste forms and then drizzle over your shake.

An apple a day really does keep the doctor away.

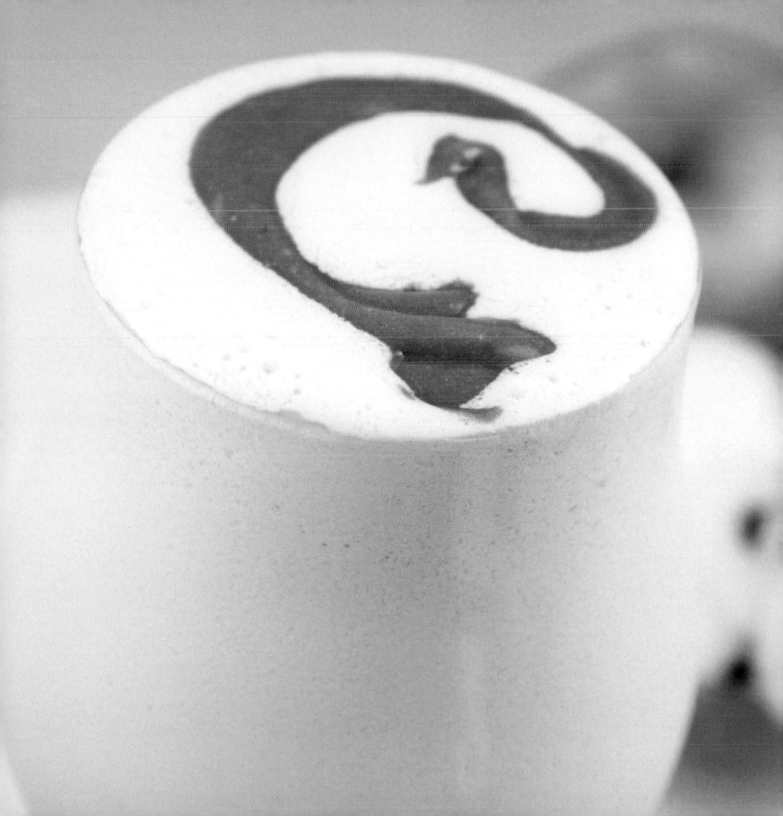

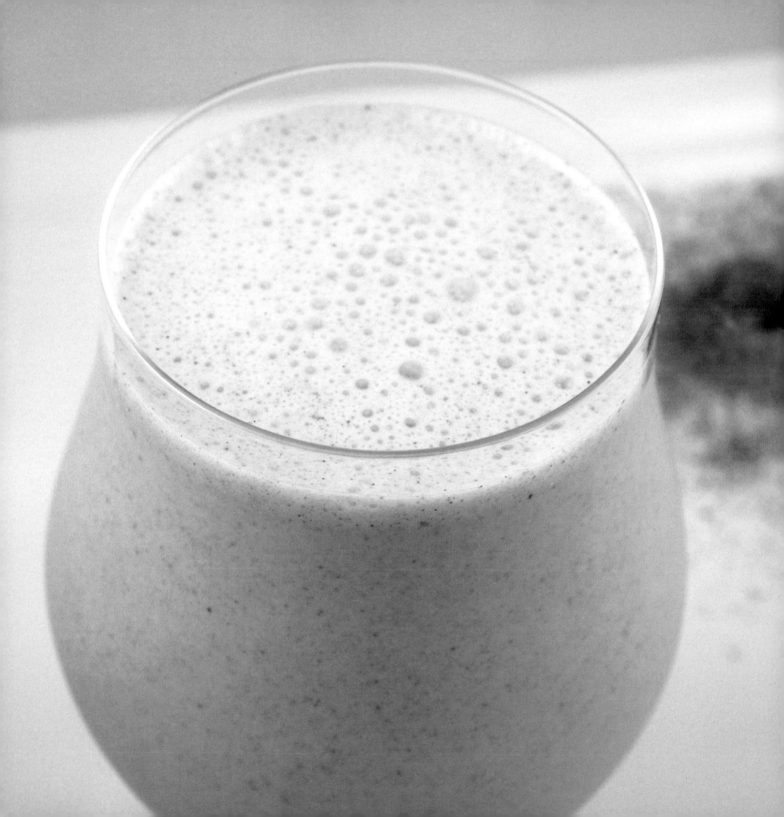

Blissful Nog

Makes 1–2 servings • Prep time: Less than 5 minutes

This is undeniably the most intensely rich and satisfying spiced nog you will ever have. It's not heavy like real eggnog or as thick as the raw-version "nut-nogs" that are around. This is just pure, satisfying pleasure.

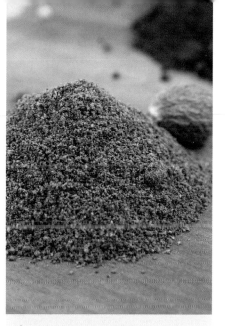

Ingredients
- 1 cup Coconut Bliss Vanilla Island
- 1 cup almond milk (or nut or seed milk of choice)
- 2 Medjool dates, pitted
- ½ teaspoon cinnamon
- ½ teaspoon nutmeg
- ½ teaspoon vanilla powder
- ⅛ teaspoon turmeric

Directions
Blend the almond milk with the dates and spices, then add your Bliss and blend to the perfect creaminess.

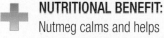

FUN FACT: In 18th-century England, just a few nutmeg nuts could create financial independence for life. It is a natural preservative.

NUTRITIONAL BENEFIT: Nutmeg calms and helps lower blood pressure. It also soothes digestive upset.

HOW TO SELECT: Select organic nutmeg, as possible, and freshly grind just prior to use.

Dates can be extremely beneficial for people suffering from stomach problems.

Café Crème

Makes 1–2 servings • Prep time: Less than 5 minutes

If I had known that this would taste so good, and that the world was looking for a way to drink their coffee with a fresh new twist, then perhaps I would have a chain of coffee stores on every street corner where people could enjoy this coconut, cold-brewed coffee delight. This is simple, delicious, and very reminiscent of America's favorite coffee shake.

Ingredients

1½ cups Coconut Bliss Vanilla Island

½ cup cold-brewed coffee concentrate

Directions

Blend Bliss and coffee on high until smooth and creamy.

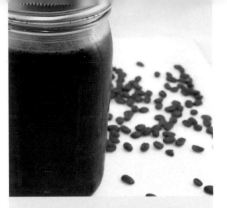

Cold-Pressed Coffee

Makes 3 cups • Stays fresh in refrigerator up to 10 days

Ingredients

½ cup freshly ground coffee

3½ cups purified water

Directions

To start, select your container. I find it easiest to use a French press, although a jar and a fine sieve will work just as well. Start with freshly roasted organic coffee beans. Coarsely grind the beans, place in container, add water, and let steep in refrigerator for 24 hours.

French press through water, or pour contents through sieve, and use.

Cold-brewed coffee contains 90% of the flavor and caffeine and only 15% of the oils and acids of hot-brewed coffee.

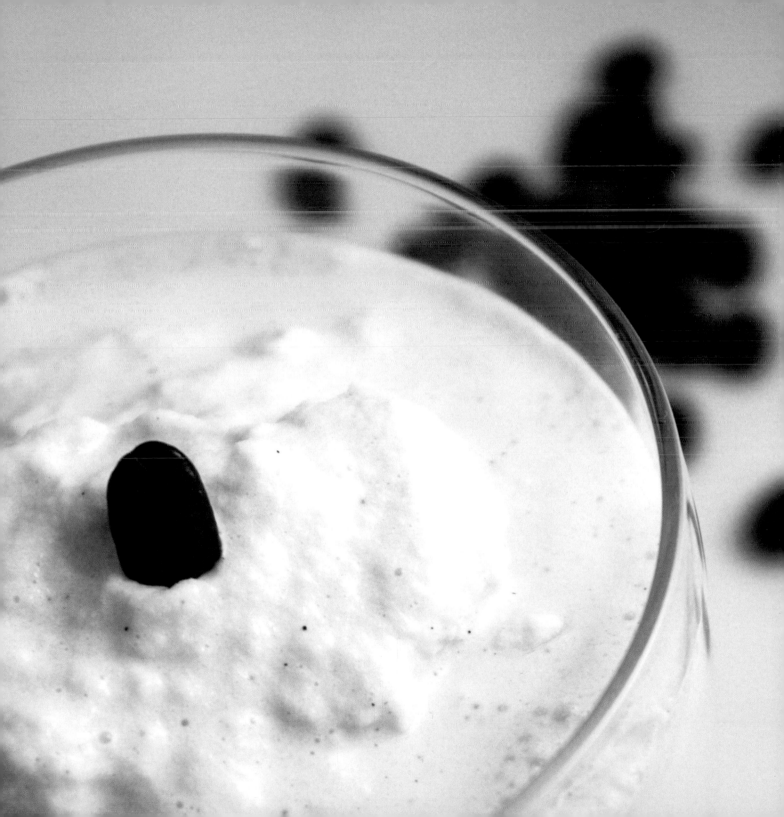

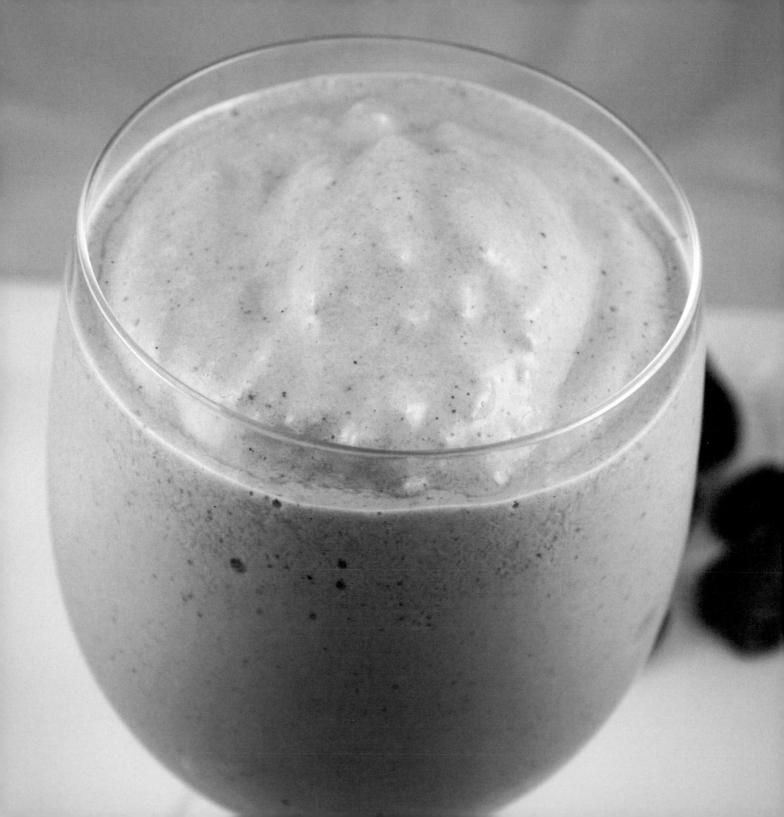

Strawberry Cream

Makes 1–2 servings • Prep time: Less than 5 minutes

When I was developing this shake, my husband proudly claimed that he was not a strawberry fan. I handed him this shake, he tasted it, and his face lit up. Then he asked for more. I guess he didn't like strawberries until he tasted Strawberry Cream. If you are using frozen strawberries, you may need to add more coconut milk.

Ingredients
1 cup Coconut Bliss Vanilla Island

1 cup coconut milk

1 cup strawberries

Directions
Blend all ingredients on high until smooth and creamy.

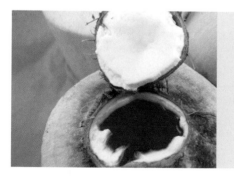

 FUN FACT: Coconut water is considered the "fluid of life" because, in a pinch, it can be used for intravenous rehydration.

 NUTRITIONAL BENEFIT: Coconut water is a natural isotonic beverage because it contains the perfect electrolyte balance.

 HOW TO SELECT: Look for clear, transparent liquid, not purplish.

Vibrant, red-colored strawberries symbolize love and spark the libido.

French Vanilla

Makes 1–2 servings • Prep time: Less than 5 minutes

Yacon syrup is a rich, molasses type of sweetener that has a distinct richness and texture. Added to a simple vanilla recipe, yacon takes the shake to a more decadent level, more like a classic French vanilla shake.

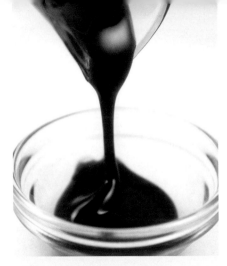

Ingredients

1½ cups Coconut Bliss Vanilla Island

½ cup brazil nut milk (or nut or seed milk of choice)

1 tablespoon yacon syrup

1 fresh vanilla bean or ½ teaspoon pure vanilla powder

1–2 Medjool dates, pitted (optional for more sweetness and richness)

Directions

Blend all ingredients on high until smooth and creamy.

FUN FACT: Related to sunflowers, yacon has large, succulent roots that have a juicy, watermelon flavor.

NUTRITIONAL BENEFIT: Yacon is glucose-free and is excellent for the low-sugar needs of diabetics.

HOW TO SELECT: Choose organic raw yacon root in syrup or dried powder.

Vanilla is an effective medicine, aphrodisiac, and insect repellent.

Dates are good for heart problems, rich in minerals, and relatively high in fiber.

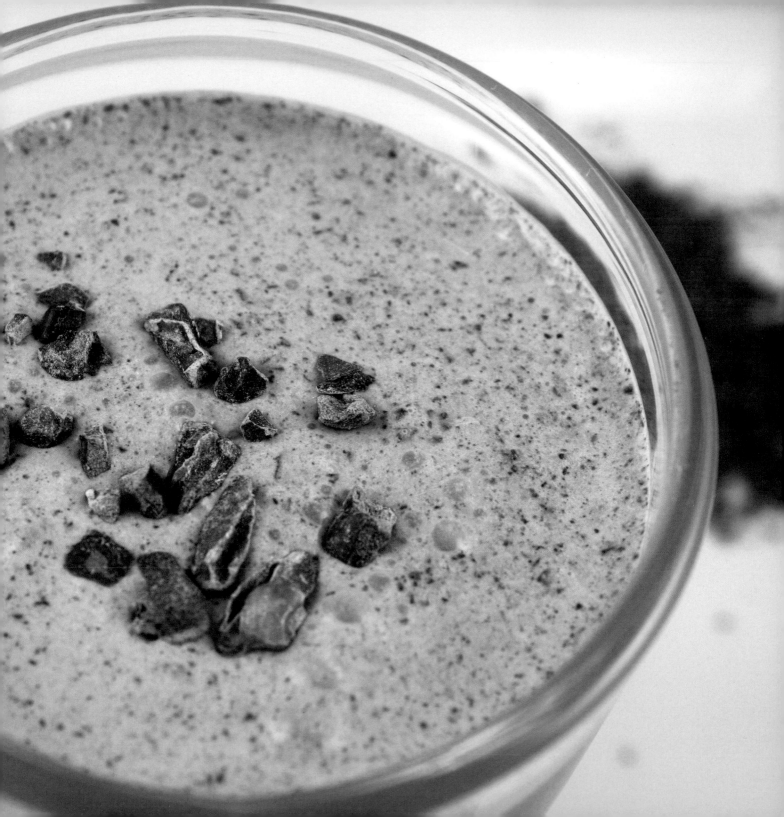

Double Chocolate Chip

Makes 1–2 servings • Prep time: Less than 5 minutes

This is as good as it gets when we are talking about decadence. This rich and chocolaty shake is loaded with happy-go-lucky chocolate bliss. Haven't you heard? Chocolate has been known to cause an uncontrollable state of bliss. I like to make it extra thick by using less nut milk and blending slightly for large chunks of chips. Then I eat it with a spoon.

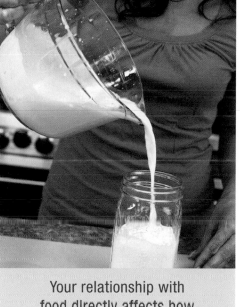

Your relationship with food directly affects how food relates to you.

Ingredients

> 1½ cups Coconut Bliss Dark Chocolate
>
> 1 cup almond milk (or nut or seed milk of choice)
>
> 2 tablespoons raw cacao nibs or dark chocolate chips

Directions

Blend all ingredients on high briefly for a thick and chunky shake or longer for a smooth and creamy one.

New York Cheesecake

Makes 1 serving • Prep time: Less than 5 minutes

This shake is like sipping on fresh cheesecake. It is so rich and satisfying, you can only drink a small amount. This would be an amazing dessert to serve at dinner parties in a beautiful snifter glass, garnished with fresh lemon or lemon zest to bring out the cheesy tang.

Ingredients

1 cup Coconut Bliss Vanilla Island

½ cup rejuvelac (see p. 39)

2 tablespoons cashew butter

2 tablespoons lemon juice

2 Medjool dates, pitted

Directions

Blend all ingredients on high until smooth and creamy.

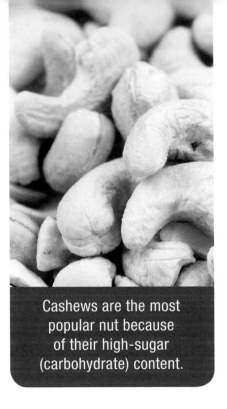

Cashews are the most popular nut because of their high-sugar (carbohydrate) content.

Sugar is the fuel of the body when taken in the correct form.

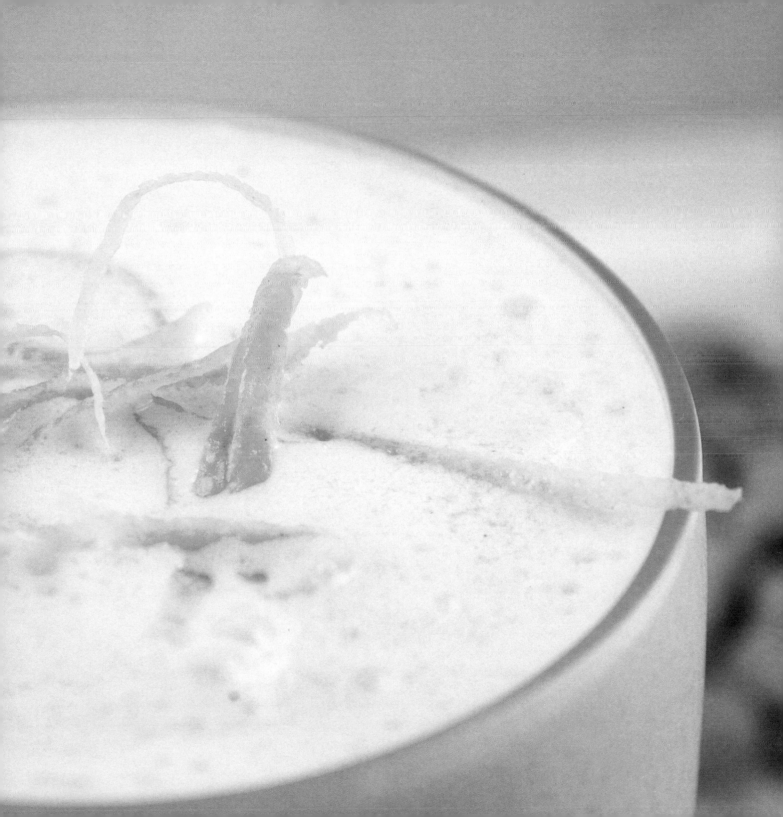

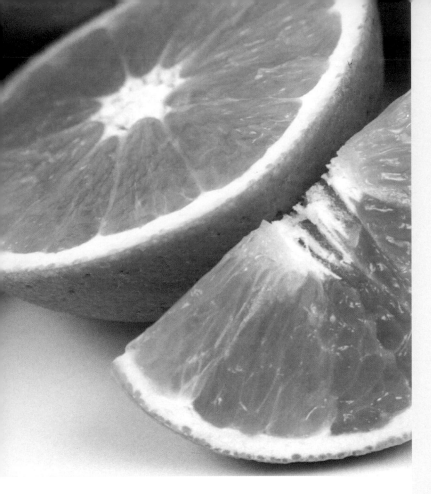

Citrus

Citrus is a goldmine for vitamin C, electrolytes, active phytochemicals, and an abundance of other vitamins and minerals that I don't want to clog your mind with. It's important to know that citrus is a low-glycemic fruit that aids the body with detoxification, acts as a beautifying agent for healthy skin and a youthful glow, and enhances cellular health. It is safe to say that citrus stimulates life. Perhaps the old adage makes sense: "An orange a day keeps the doctor at bay."

- **Orange:** The classic, juicy orange comes in many varieties, such as Valencia, Navel, and Jaffa.
- **Blood orange:** These stunning oranges have a bright-red pulp with very intense and delicious flavor.
- **Cara cara:** This is an extra-sweet orange with pinkish-red pulp.
- **Tangerine:** Tangerines are small, classic, seeded fruits with a yummy sweet flavor.
- **Minneola tangelo:** This is an easy-to-peel, juicy tangerine.
- **Satsuma mandarin:** Satsumas are thick and bumpy skinned, but have delicate, sweet centers.
- **Clementine:** This mini-tangerine is like delicate candy.
- **Lemon:** Lemon is a tart, alkalizing fruit. The major varieties are Lisbon and Eureka.
- **Meyer lemon:** Originally a cross between a lemon and an orange, a Meyer is a sweeter lemon with golden pulp.
- **Lime:** This is a small, green, tart, and highly alkalizing fruit.
- **Grapefruit:** The round, plump, juicy, and slightly bitter fruit comes in many varieties and shades of pink and yellow.
- **Pummelo:** Pummelo, also called Chinese grapefruit, is large and pulpy.

The juice quality of all citrus fruits improves during the season. The longer the fruit stays on the tree, the better it gets.

Supercharged Bliss

You've heard of superfoods and are learning more about what they are each day. Now, you are going to incorporate them into your diet by making mouth-watering shakes that will heal your body and make your health soar to the next level. You may add superfoods to any food, drink, or smoothie, but right now you are going to integrate them into your life with Supercharged Bliss. Ready for take off?

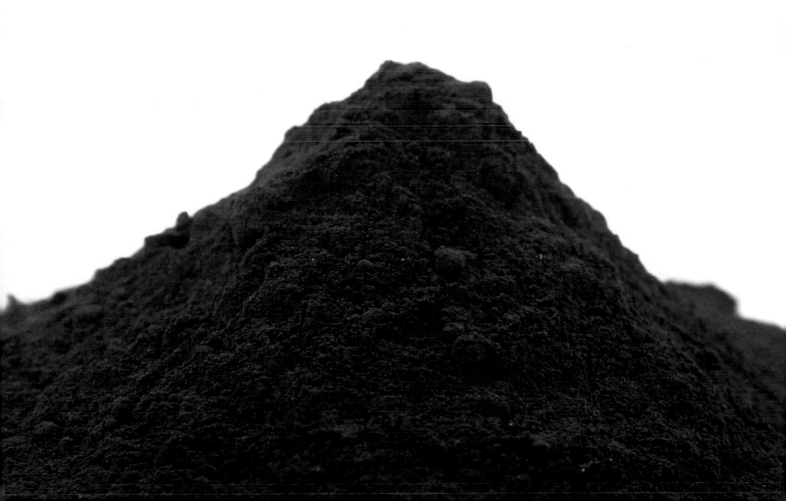

Goji Mojo

Makes 1–2 servings • Prep time: Less than 5 minutes

Goji berries are the most widely spread superfood in the marketplace. The dried berries are available in packages and bulk, and sometimes you can find them in powdered form. You can use any form of goji berry that you like. I'm trying to grow my own now, so perhaps I will be making this fresh next time. The taste is mild and sweet. This shake is smooth and delicious and has an anti-aging effect because of its supercharged berry.

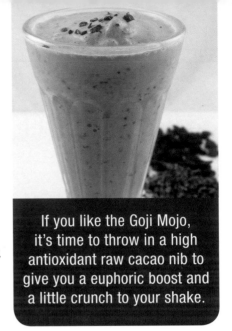

If you like the Goji Mojo, it's time to throw in a high antioxidant raw cacao nib to give you a euphoric boost and a little crunch to your shake.

Ingredients

1½ cups Coconut Bliss Vanilla Island

½ cup almond milk (or nut or seed milk of choice)

½ cup rejuvelac (see p. 39)

2 tablespoons goji berries

2 Medjool dates, pitted

1 cup ice cubes (optional)

Directions

Blend all ingredients on high until smooth and creamy.

Goji Mojo Chip

Follow the directions for a Goji Mojo shake, then add 2 tablespoons of raw cacao nibs or dark chocolate chips. Blend until chopped and incorporated.

. . . .

Goji berries can keep you young by promoting human growth hormone production.

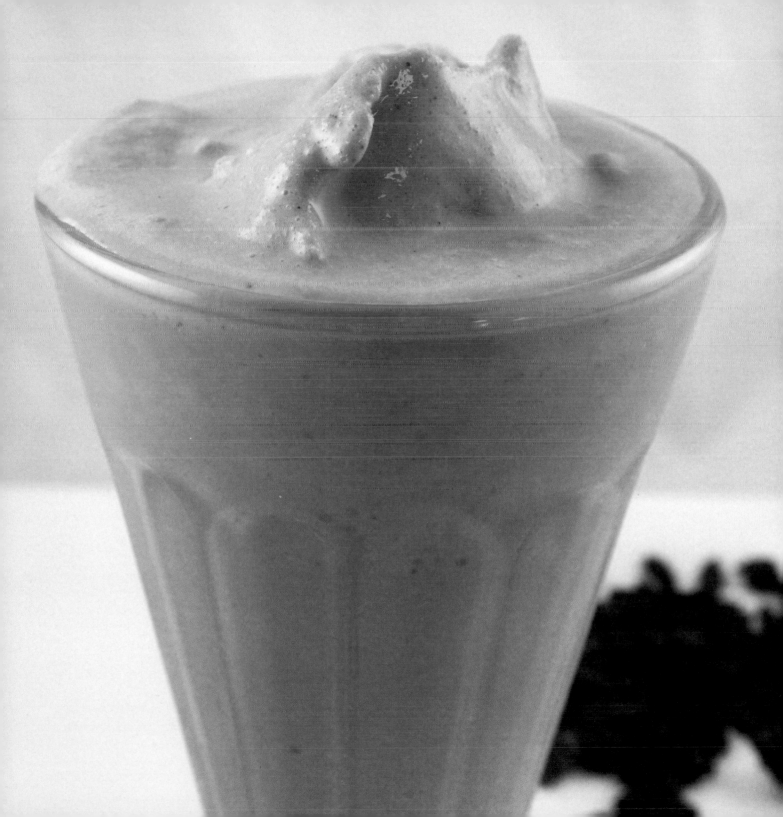

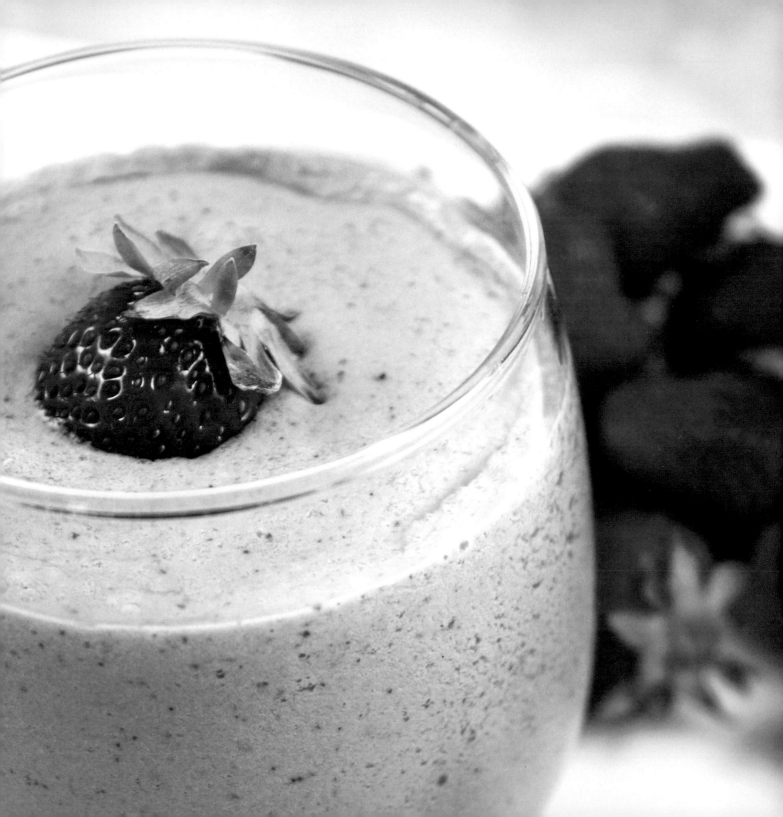

Strawberry Recharge

Makes 1–2 servings • Prep time: Less than 5 minutes

Camu camu is a delicious, tart, berry-like powder that adds a huge boost of vitamin C to anything you eat. It's great for an energy boost, immune support, or just a little sparkle in your radiant face. It's so yummy and highly nutritious, you can add it to any shake or smoothie, but I like it best with strawberries and hazelnut milk—a combination that I found works really well.

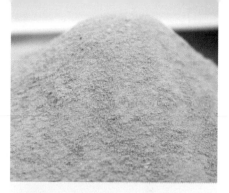

FUN FACT: The size of a large cherry, a camu camu berry provides 30 times more vitamin C than an orange.

NUTRITIONAL BENEFIT: Camu camu helps with depression by supporting serotonin levels, which elevates the mood.

HOW TO SELECT: Camu camu is only available in powdered form in the U.S.

Ingredients

- 1 cup Coconut Bliss Vanilla Island
- ½ cup hazelnut milk (or nut or seed milk of choice)
- 1 cup fresh strawberries
- 2 teaspoons camu camu powder
- 1 cup ice cubes (optional)

Directions

Blend all ingredients on high until smooth and creamy.

Camu camu is a potent botanical support for a strong immune system and balanced moods.
It is ranked among the top 5 most effective healing plants.

Bee My Honey

Makes 1–2 servings • Prep time: Less than 5 minutes

It is said that a quarter teaspoon of royal jelly gives you all the minerals you need for the day. One thing's for sure, adding royal jelly to a Blissful shake with fresh alkalizing lemon juice and honey makes a tangy, creamy, celebrated treat.

Ingredients

1 cup Coconut Bliss Vanilla Island

1 cup almond milk (or nut or seed milk of choice)

¼ cup freshly squeezed lemon juice

1 tablespoon raw honey

¼ teaspoon royal jelly

1 cup ice cubes (optional)

Directions
Blend all ingredients on high until smooth and creamy.

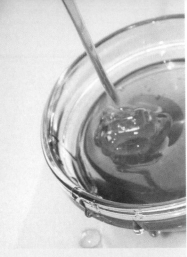

FUN FACT: Honey never spoils. Plus, it would take about 1 ounce of honey to fuel a honeybee's flight around the world.

NUTRITIONAL BENEFIT: Honey is the only food that includes all the substances necessary to sustain life, including water.

HOW TO SELECT: Choose raw, unheated honey, preferably wild.

Raw honey is the richest source of healing enzymes.

Royal jelly can help strengthen your immune system and give you more energy and an overall youthful glow.

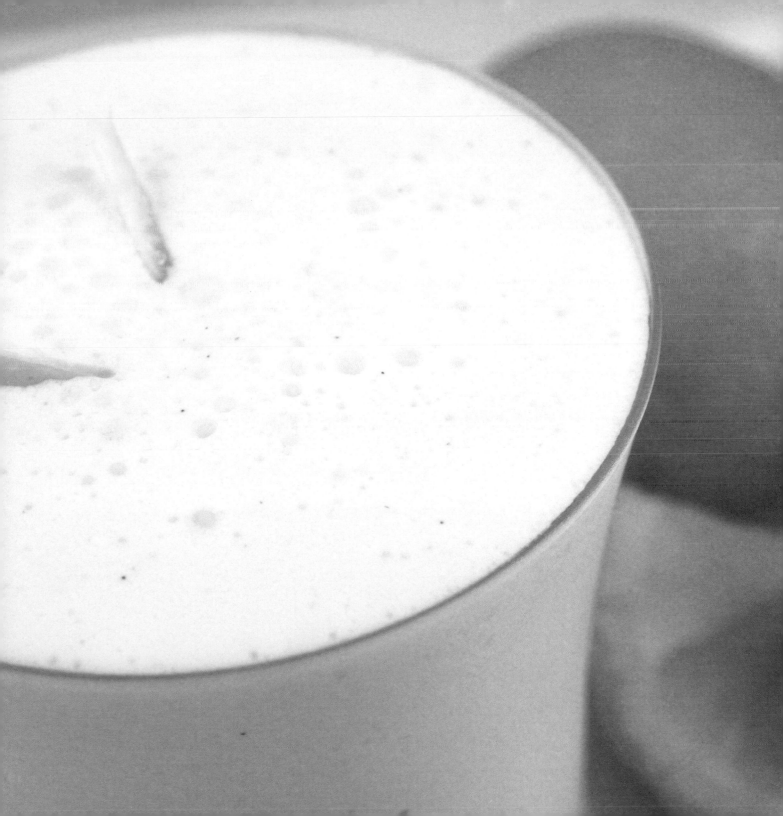

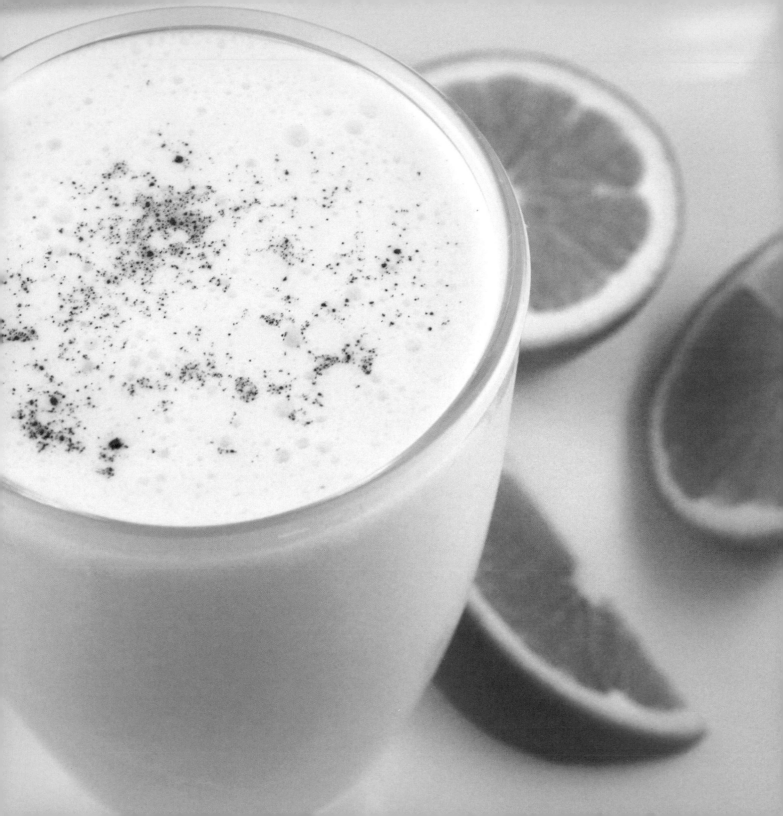

Creamsicle Bliss

Makes 1–2 servings • Prep time: 5 minutes (or longer if juicing your oranges fresh)

I was craving a Creamsicle bar one day and made this combination. I did a tasting of it at a health-food market, and the maca created such a buzz that the market claimed they sold more maca that day than they had in the last 3 months. It turned out that people had heard of maca, but just didn't know how to consume it. Thus the magic of Supercharged Bliss!

Ingredients

1 cup Coconut Bliss Vanilla Island

1½ cups freshly squeezed orange juice

½ teaspoon maca powder

Dash of pure vanilla powder

Directions

Blend all ingredients on high until smooth and creamy.

FUN FACT: Vanilla is an orchid known throughout history for its aphrodisiac qualities.

NUTRITIONAL BENEFIT: Vanilla has a calming and soothing effect that can induce a sense of euphoria.

HOW TO SELECT: Choose raw, organic vanilla powder and store it in a cool, dry place.

Maca can enhance libido and sexual function.

Cranberry Chip

Makes 1–2 servings • Prep time: Less than 5 minutes

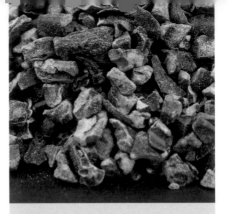

This shake is such an amazing combination that for a while I found myself making it nightly for my daughter. She couldn't get enough of it. She loves the combination of cranberries and chocolate, and the uplifting effect gives her the energy to do her homework in pure bliss.

Ingredients

1½ cups Coconut Bliss Vanilla Island

1 cup almond milk (or nut or seed milk of choice)

½ cup cranberries

2 Medjool dates, pitted

1–2 tablespoons cacao nibs

Directions

Blend all ingredients except cacao on high until smooth and creamy. Add cacao nibs and blend until they are chopped and incorporated.

FUN FACT: Eating raw cacao increases the same brain chemicals that we have when excited, happy, or sexually aroused.

NUTRITIONAL BENEFIT: Cacao is high in flavonoids, which help promote cardiovascular health.

HOW TO SELECT: Select raw cacao, not cocoa powder.

The cranberry is a powerhouse of antioxidants, topping the charts next to the beloved blueberry.

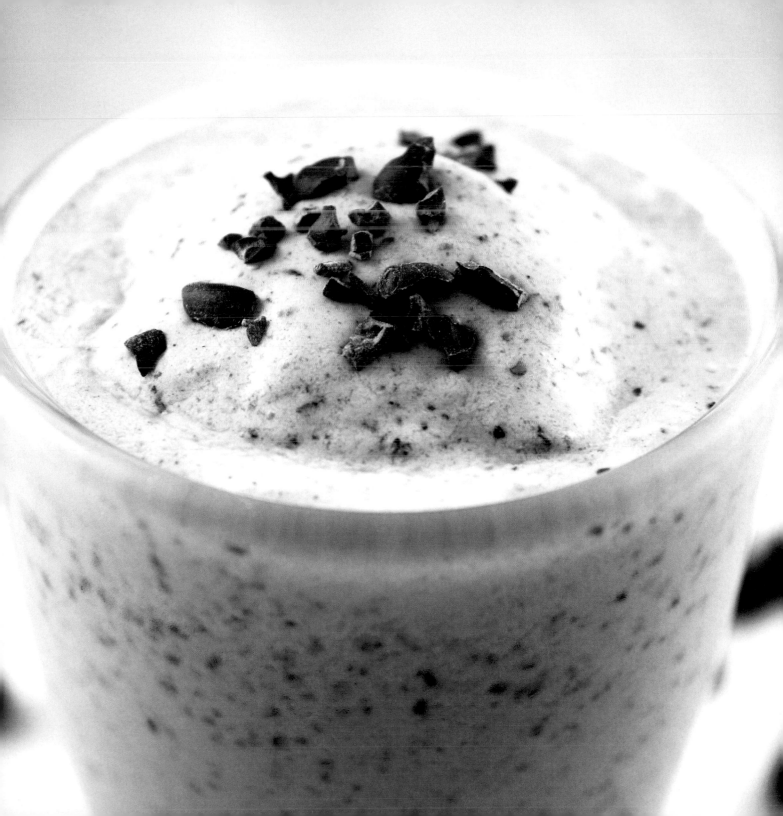

Southern Comfort

Makes 1 2 servings • Prep time: Less than 5 minutes

If you like creamy comfort foods with a maple twist, you'll like this shake that is sweet and reminiscent of the south. Add a little raw Peruvian mesquite pod and supercharge your shake to a sweet and nutritional level, enjoying the full potential of this wild-crafted pod.

Ingredients

 1 cup Coconut Bliss Vanilla Island

 ½ cup almond milk (or nut or seed milk of choice)

 2 tablespoons pure organic maple syrup

 1 teaspoon mesquite pod flour

Directions

Blend all ingredients on high until smooth and creamy.

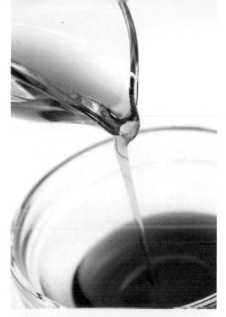

FUN FACT: It takes 30 to 50 gallons of sap to make one gallon of maple syrup.

NUTRITIONAL BENEFIT: Maple syrup benefits the immune system, supports reproductive health, and provides special benefits for men.

HOW TO SELECT: Choose B-grade maple syrup for its rich flavor and high mineral content.

Sweet Cherry Love

Makes 1–2 servings • Prep time: Less than 5 minutes

Inspired by an edible facial mask I make with Montmorency cherries and tocotrienols that leaves my skin soft, silky, and sweet smelling, this milkshake beautifies from within. The tocotrienols give a big boost of vitamin E.

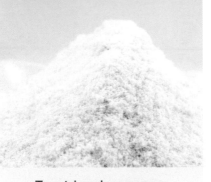

Tocotrienols possess powerful antioxidant, anticancer, and cholesterol-lowering properties.

Ingredients

1 cup Coconut Bliss Vanilla Island

1 cup coconut milk

1 cup sweet cherries

2 tablespoons tocotrienols powder

Directions

Blend all ingredients on high until smooth and creamy.

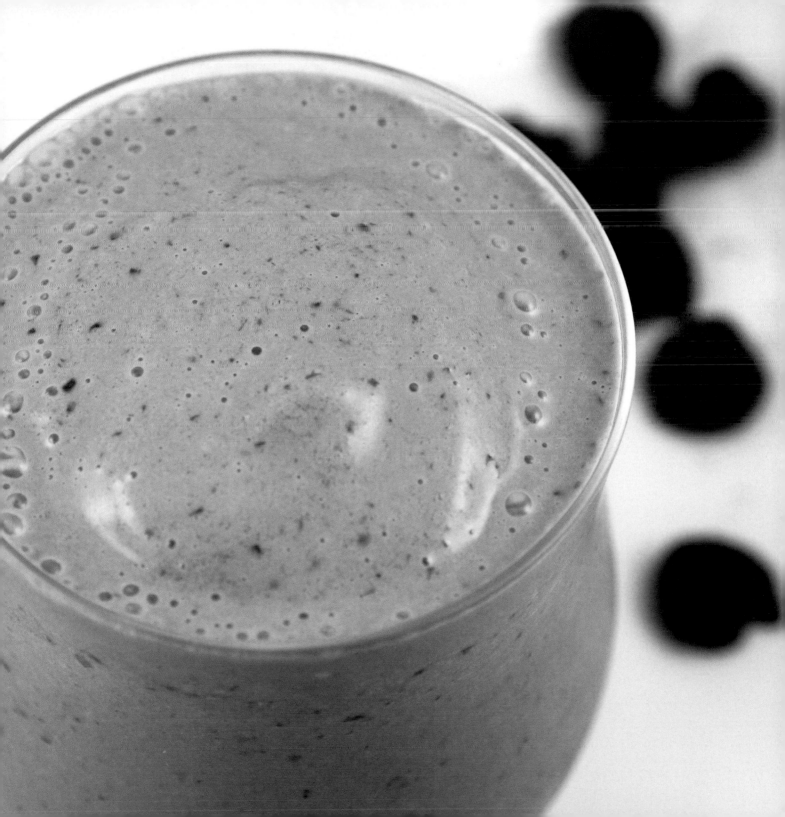

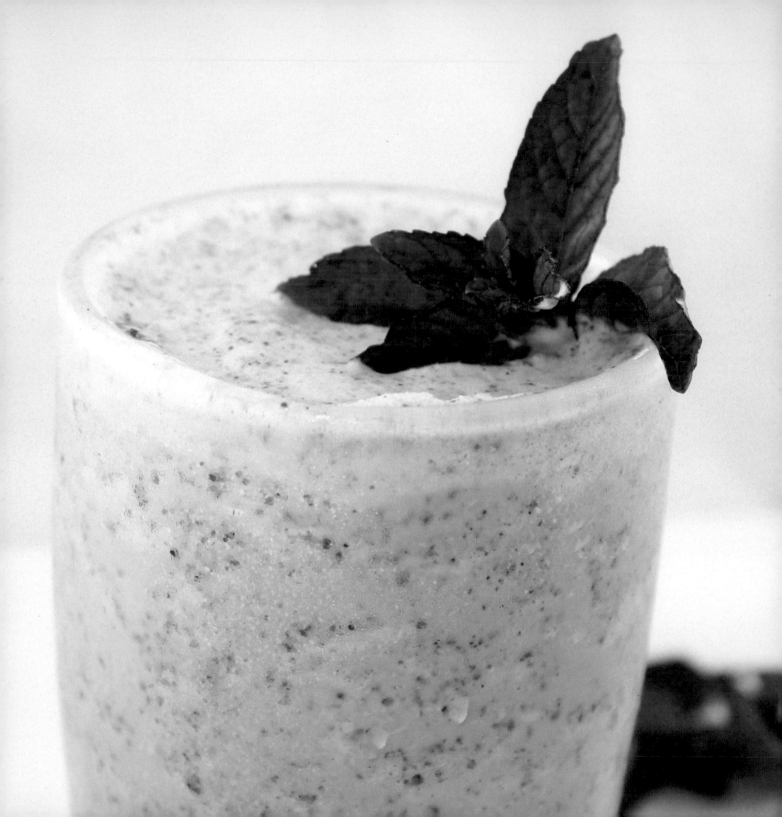

Mint Chocolate Chip

Makes 1–2 servings • Prep time: Less than 5 minutes

I don't know anyone who doesn't love the minty coolness of mint chocolate chip ice cream. This refreshing, classic shake is sure to win your heart and become a mainstay in your blissful life. It is not only delicious, but it is supercharged for ultimate nutrition.

Ingredients

1½ cups Coconut Bliss Vanilla Island

1 cup almond milk (or nut or seed milk of choice)

12 mint leaves (or 4–6 drops of organic peppermint oil)

½ teaspoon vanilla extract

2 Medjool dates, pitted

1 teaspoon spirulina

2 tablespoons raw cacao nibs

1 cup of ice (optional)

Directions

Place all ingredients except raw cacao nibs in blender and blend until smooth. Add cacao nibs and ice cubes and blend until ground. Garnish with a mint leaf.

Vanilla Malted

Makes 1–2 servings • Prep time: Less than 5 minutes

Newly rediscovered in the marketplace, maca root is great for hormonal balance in both men and women. It has been revered as a key to a healthy sex life for many years. This yummy vanilla shake is supercharged with this Peruvian root, which adds a malt-like flavor.

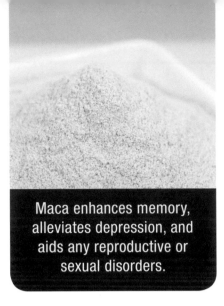

Maca enhances memory, alleviates depression, and aids any reproductive or sexual disorders.

Ingredients

1½ cups Coconut Bliss Vanilla Island

1 cup almond milk (or nut or seed milk of choice)

1 teaspoon pure vanilla powder

1½ teaspoons maca powder

2 Medjool dates, pitted

Directions
Blend all ingredients on high until smooth and creamy.

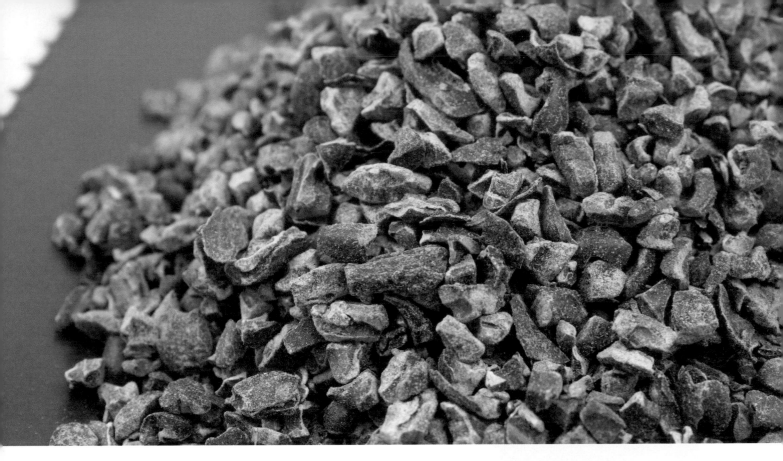

Raw Chocolate—
The Bliss Chemical

Chocolate is known as the "food of the gods." It contains anandamide, which is a neurotransmitter found in the human brain known to cause an overall feeling of joy. The word "anandamide" is derived from the Sanskrit word *ananda* meaning "bliss."

Raw cacao can:

- Increase overall health.
- Lower depression and stress.
- Increase mental alertness and power.
- Decrease appetite.
- Create a youthful and playful energy.

"Save the Earth—it's the only planet with chocolate." ~Author unknown

Pure Decadence

Why not? I mean if it tastes good and won't cause you pain, I say a little indulgence is good for the soul.

These milkshakes are designed for your pure pleasure and, by the way, they have nutritional value as well. They are a rich and satisfying alternative to the high-calorie, high fat milkshakes that we all grew up on. Remember what I always say: "If you are not enjoying your healing process, then you are not healing."

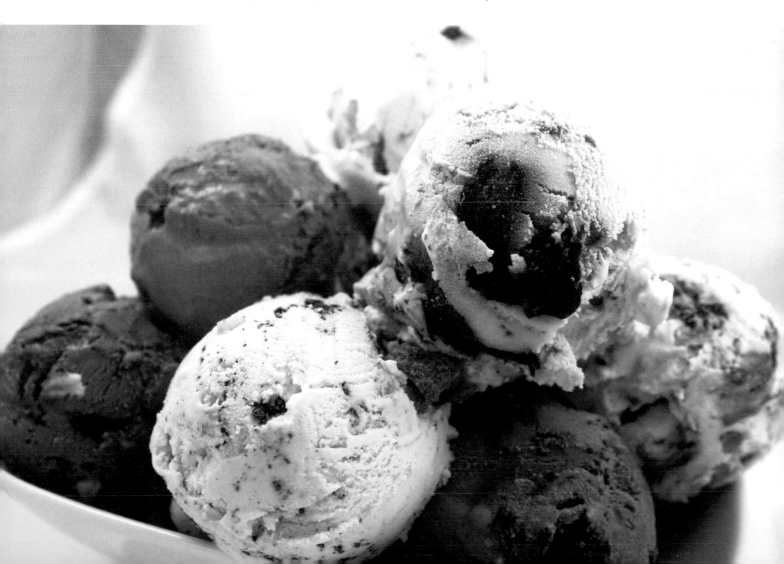

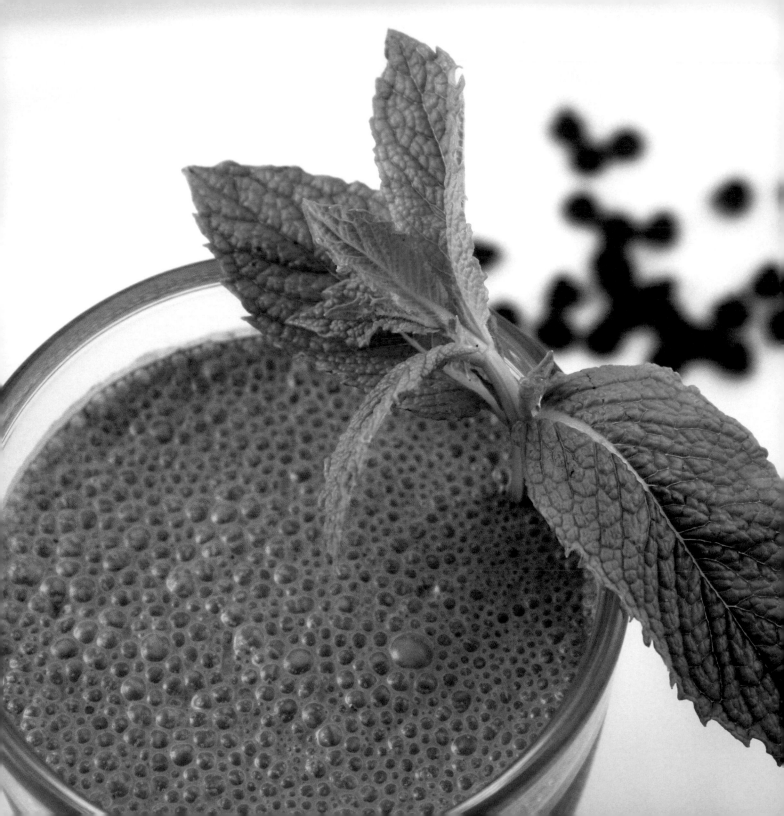

Minty Fudge

Makes 1–2 servings • Prep time: Less than 5 minutes

Oh, this is a good one. Really yummy! I've made it with spirulina and without. It doesn't affect the taste, it just changes the color a little. So, if you can add all the benefits of a superfood without compromising joy, then I say, "why not?" If you prefer, you may substitute fresh organic peppermint oil for fresh mint, but use only a few drops because it is very strong.

Ingredients

1½ cups Coconut Bliss Dark Chocolate

12 fresh mint leaves (or 4–6 drops of organic peppermint oil)

1 cup almond milk (or nut or seed milk of choice)

2 teaspoons raw cacao powder

1 teaspoon spirulina (optional)

Directions

Blend all ingredients on high until smooth and creamy.

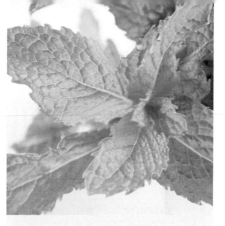

FUN FACT: Mint was once so valued, it was used as a form of payment.

NUTRITIONAL BENEFIT: Mint helps relieve migraine headaches as well as facial or other muscular tension.

HOW TO SELECT: Choose fresh, bright-green mint leaves.

Mint mixed with cacao creates a magical concoction. Both foods enhance each other's medicinal properties.

Eat more spirulina for a glowing complexion.

Cherry Vanilla Chocolate Chip

Makes 1–2 servings • Prep time: Less than 5 minutes

I'm a big cherry fan. There is something special about this particular fruit to me. I had to control myself so that I wouldn't make too many shake recipes with cherries. This particular one stood out as crazy decadence—in other words, "Oh my, this is good."

Ingredients

1½ cups Coconut Bliss Vanilla Island

1 cup almond milk (or nut or seed milk of choice)

1 cup pitted cherries

1 teaspoon vanilla extract

2 tablespoons cacao nibs

Directions

Blend all ingredients except cacao on high until smooth and creamy. Then add cacao nibs and blend until they are chopped and incorporated.

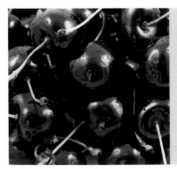

 FUN FACT: The bark and stems of wild cherries smell like almonds.

 NUTRITIONAL BENEFIT: Cherries help regulate sleep, aid with jet lag, prevent memory loss, and delay the aging process.

 HOW TO SELECT: Look for plump, dark-purplish cherries.

Cherries are one of the best food sources of iron.

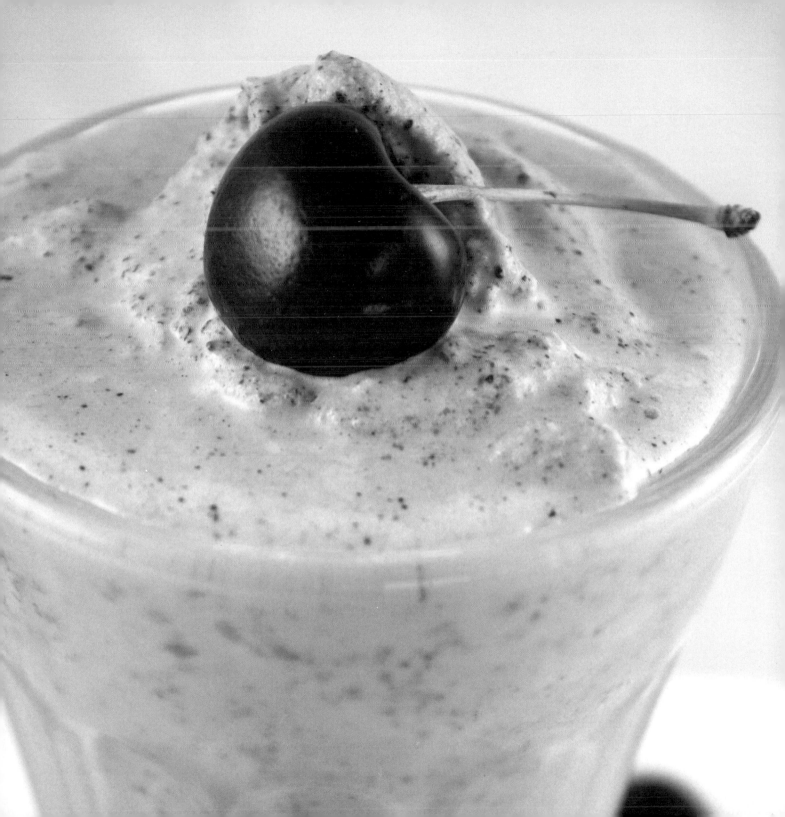

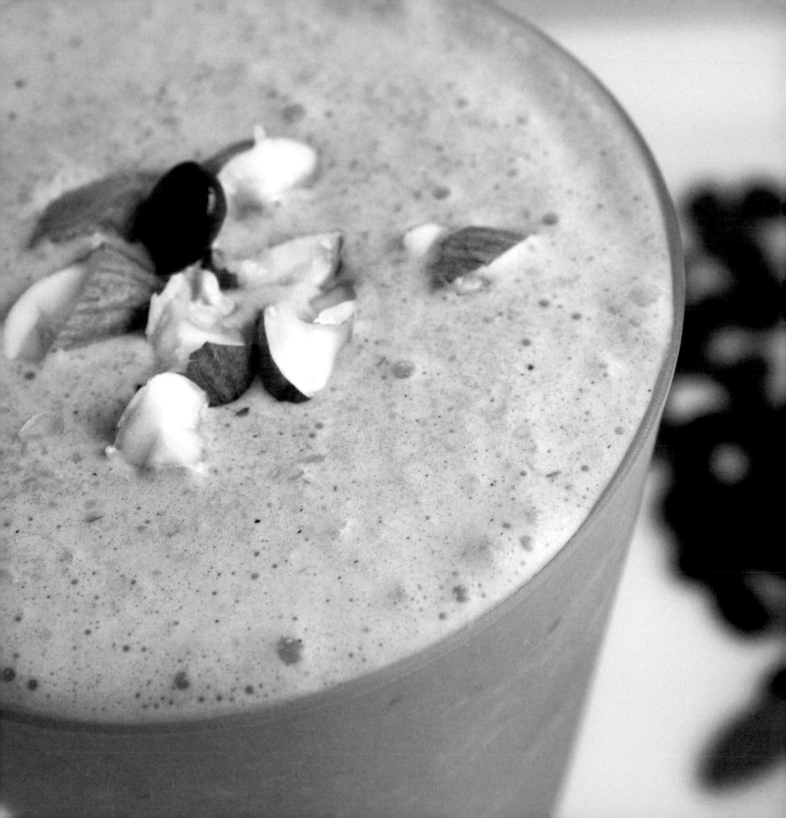

Mocha Almond Fudge

Makes 1–2 servings • Prep time: Less than 5 minutes

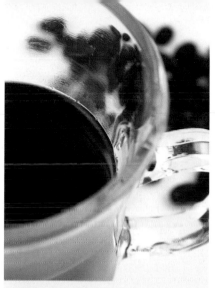

This shake was inspired by one of my favorite flavors at the ice cream shop. Chocolate mixed with coffee and almonds for a slight crunch in every sip combine to make a super-special treat that adds a bit of bliss to your life.

Ingredients

1½ cups Coconut Bliss Dark Chocolate

½ cup cold-pressed coffee concentrate (see p. 92)

½ cup almond milk (or nut or seed milk of choice)

1–2 tablespoons raw almonds

Directions

Blend all ingredients except almonds on high until smooth and creamy. Add almonds and blend with a pulse action to chop and incorporate.

Top with chopped almonds.

 FUN FACT: The coffee bean is actually a berry. For many, it is the largest source of antioxidants in their diet.

 NUTRITIONAL BENEFIT: Cold-pressed coffee is 67% less acidic than hot-brewed coffee.

$ HOW TO SELECT: Choose organic coffee beans.

Cold-pressed coffee takes a little more time to prepare, but the low acid and mild flavor make it worth the effort.

Creamy Caramel Swirl

Makes 1–2 servings • Prep time: 5 minutes

This shake is a double delight—a thick, caramel-flavored shake with a drizzle of healthful caramel sauce. I like to double the caramel sauce recipe for double the fun. Make a large batch and you've got a delicious caramel dip for your fresh fruit.

Ingredients

- 1½ cups Coconut Bliss Vanilla Island
- 1 cup almond milk (or nut or seed milk of choice)
- 1 tablespoon lucuma powder
- 2 Medjool dates, pitted

Directions

Blend all ingredients on high until smooth and creamy.

Caramel Sauce

Ingredients

- 1 teaspoon lucuma powder
- 1 teaspoon maple syrup

Directions

Mix together in a small bowl or ramekin until a caramel paste forms. Drizzle over milkshake.

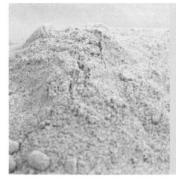

 FUN FACT: Lucuma is a tropical fruit grown in Peru and Chile. It has a green skin and yellow flesh. When dried and powdered, it makes a wonderful low-sugar sweetener with a rich, maple flavor.

 NUTRITIONAL BENEFIT: Lucuma is low in acid and rich with carbohydrates, fiber, vitamins, minerals, and beta-carotene.

 HOW TO SELECT: Powdered lucuma should have a bright yellow color.

Lucuma powder is an incredible source of beta-carotene, which is a great support for eye health.

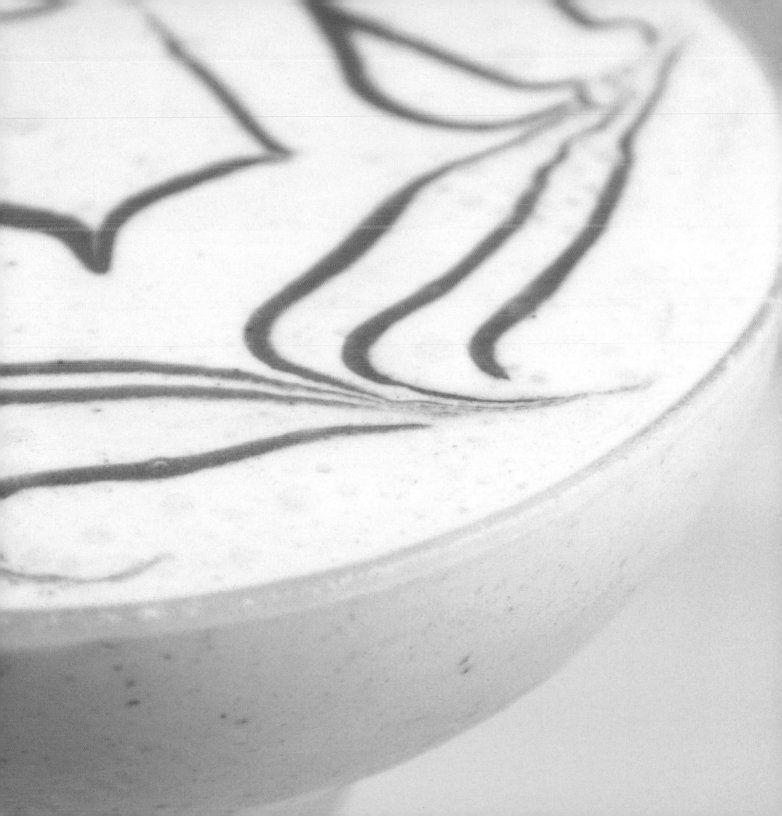

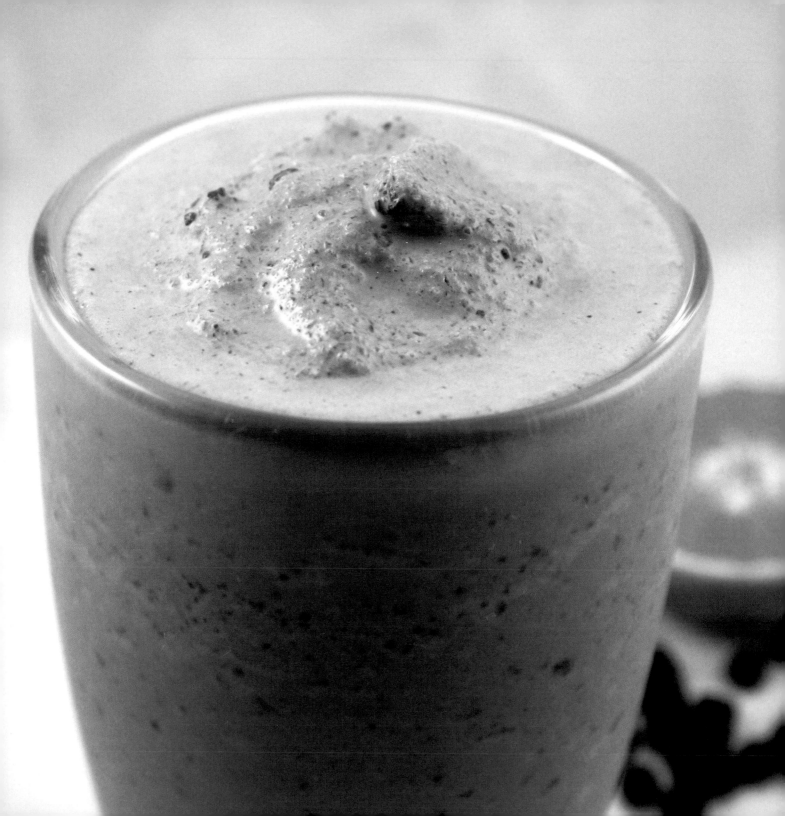

Chocolate Orange Chip

Makes 1–2 servings • Prep time: Less than 5 minutes (or longer if juicing your oranges fresh)

Everything goes well with chocolate, but orange with chocolate is a classic temptress kind of delicious. There is something sexy about this combination, and when I serve it at home, the reaction I get from its elegant flavors proves it.

Ingredients

- 1½ cups Coconut Bliss Dark Chocolate
- 1 cup freshly squeezed orange juice
- 1–2 tablespoons cacao nibs or dark chocolate chips

Directions

Blend orange juice and Bliss on high until creamy and smooth. Add chocolate and blend until chopped and incorporated.

For a burst of flavor, add orange zest to your shakes. Orange peel contains limonene, a very potent natural chemical that helps the body eliminate carcinogens.

Red Velvet

Makes 1–2 servings • Prep time: 5 minutes (or longer if juicing your beets fresh)

The original red velvet cake was made with red food coloring and a small amount of chocolate. It was considered a poor man's chocolate cake because the price of cacao was so high, it was wise to use it sparingly. The red added a rich color. Well, the same is true for beet juice. If I were you, I would throw the beet greens into the blender as well; it makes for a more supercharged vitamin boost and does not change the flavor.

Ingredients

1½ cups Coconut Bliss Dark Chocolate

½ cup almond milk (or nut or seed milk of choice)

1 cup fresh-pressed beet juice

½ frozen banana

3–4 leaves of beet greens (optional)

Directions
Blend all ingredients on high until smooth and creamy.

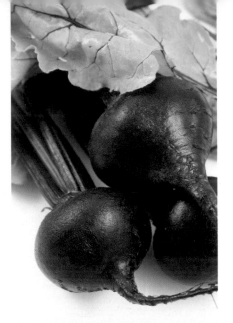

FUN FACT: Beets are in the same family as bougainvillea, carnations, and Venus flytraps.

NUTRITIONAL BENEFIT: Beets help defeat cancer, anemia, and urinary tract infections.

HOW TO SELECT: Choose beets with firm, smooth skins and non-wilted leaves, if still attached. Smaller ones are more tender.

Cognitive brain function is dependent on natural-sugar foods.

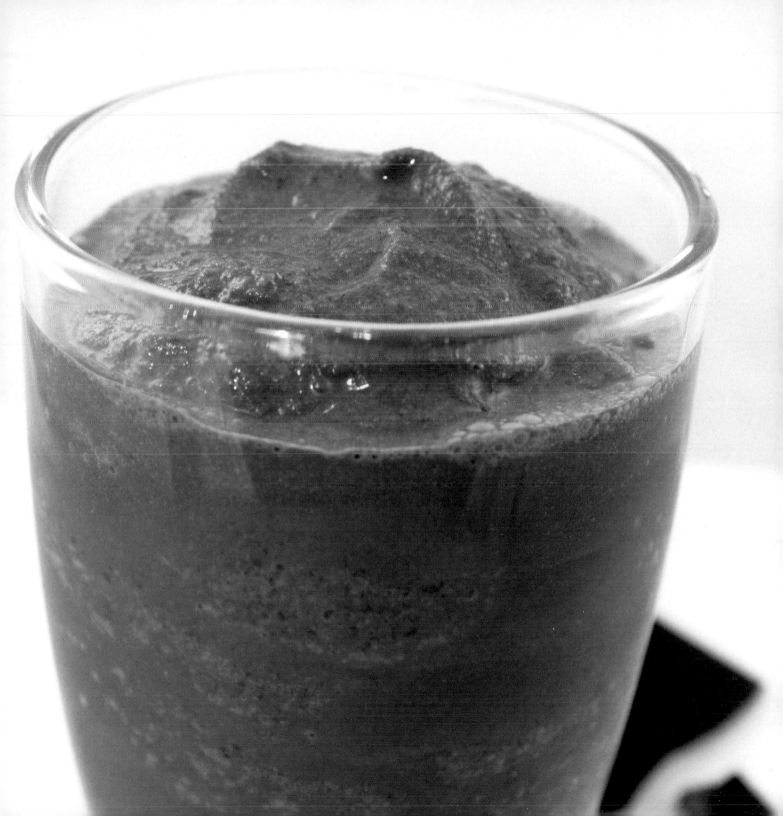

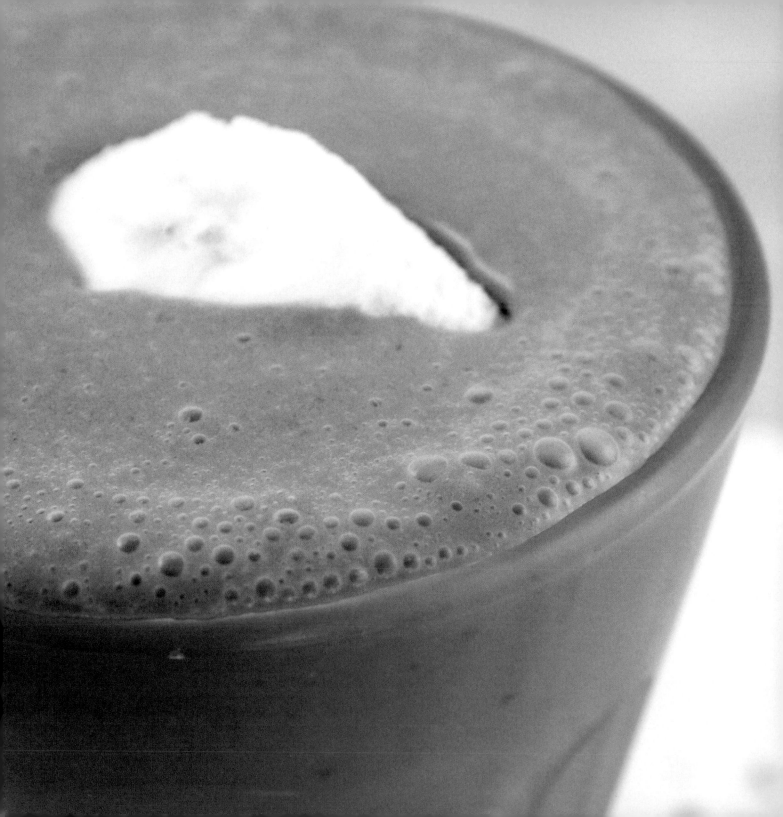

Chocolate-Covered Banana

Makes 1–2 servings • Prep time: Less than 5 minutes

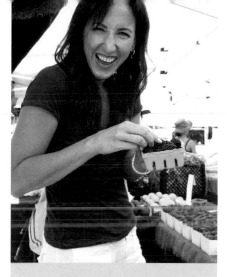

Struggling with diet inhibits life.

The first time I made this simple shake, it disappeared from the kitchen. Then I made it again, and it walked off with someone else. I finally had the brilliance to photograph it quickly before it vanished, and it was gone, again. I came to find out that one of my helpers (who never liked chocolate before) kept pouring it into a coffee cup to disguise it so that she could enjoy it all by herself. It's that good!

Ingredients

1½ cups Coconut Bliss Dark Chocolate

1 cup almond milk (or nut or seed milk of choice)

1 frozen banana

Directions

Blend all ingredients on high until smooth and creamy.

Coconut Almond Fudge

Makes 1–2 servings • Prep time: 5–10 minutes

Even I am surprised when something this delicious isn't considered a "know no." It may not be filled with produce or superfoods, but it is certainly Naked—just the way we like it!

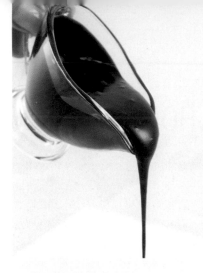

Ingredients

- 1½ cups Coconut Bliss Naked Coconut
- 1 cup coconut milk
- 2 Medjool dates, pitted
- 2 teaspoons shaved coconut
- 1–2 tablespoons chopped raw almonds

Directions

Blend all ingredients except almonds on high until smooth and creamy. Add almonds and blend with a pulse action to chop and incorporate. Top with fudge drizzle and chopped almonds.

Fudge Drizzle

Ingredients

- 1 tablespoon agave nectar (or maple syrup)
- 1 tablespoon raw cacao powder

Directions

Mix together in a small bowl or ramekin until a creamy fudge forms and then drizzle over milkshake.

> A 1.4-ounce piece of raw cacao has the same amount of caffeine as an 8-ounce cup of decaffeinated coffee.

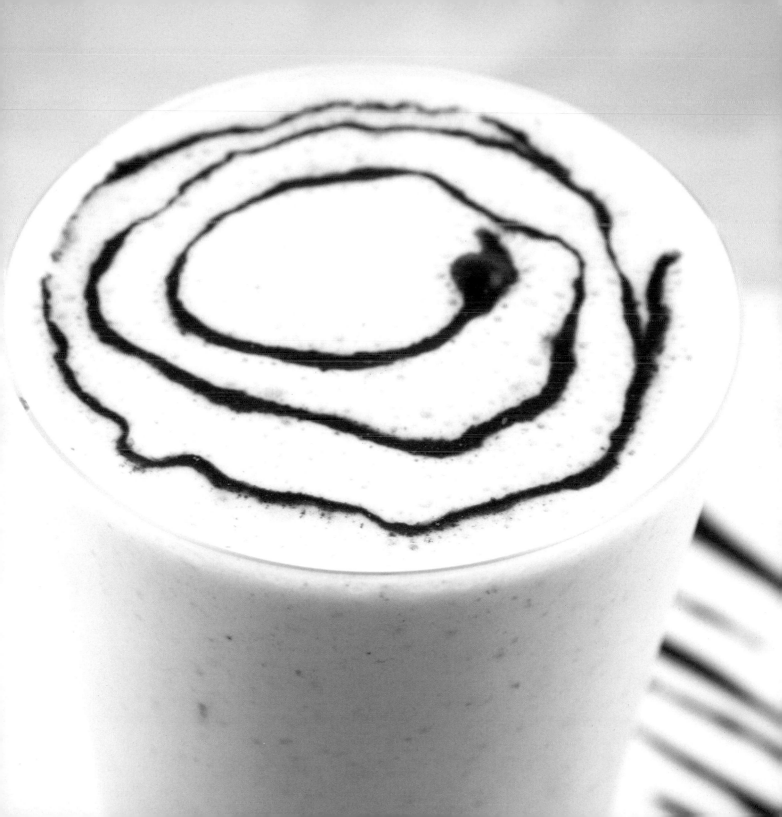

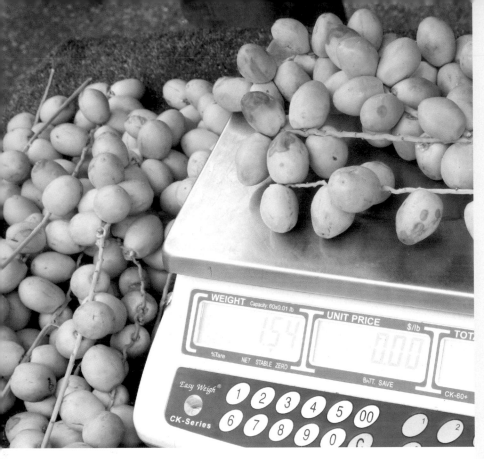

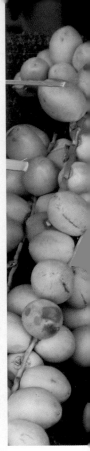

Medjool dates are the largest and most popular variety and are easily found in grocery stores or specialty shops. They are large, soft and creamy, incredibly sweet dates. They are considered the "Cadillac of dates."

Deglet Noor dates are the most commonly sold date in the U.S. It is a long, thin, semi-dry, and "thready" textured date. It is an orange-brown, somewhat chewy, moderately sweet fruit that is used in all sorts of date recipes and candies.

Barhi dates are little round, candy-like fruits with thick, caramel-flavored flesh. They may be found online or in farmers' markets. (They are pictured here in a fresh-picked, unripened state.)

Khadrawy dates are soft, reddish brown, and slightly wrinkled. They have more moisture and less sugar than some other date varieties. They are sweet with a caramel-like inside texture.

Halawi dates are the original date brought over from the Middle East for cultivation. They are dark gold, soft, wrinkled, very flavorful, but not too sweet.

Zahidi dates (golden dates) are grown primarily in the Middle East. They are an oval, brownish-yellow, semi-dry, moderately sweet date. Date sugar comes from this variety.

Getting to Know Your Date

Dates are sweet, tender, and loving to the body. They provide a natural sugar that is high in carbohydrates, which give you instant energy. As a great source of iron, B vitamins, and amino acids, dates are an excellent, sweet substitute for sugar in a Naked lifestyle. They are rich in minerals that our bodies need to function well.

Another advantage of dates is that they keep for a long time. When refrigerated they will keep for up to a year. Make sure to store them in an airtight container to preserve their moisture. Because of dates' high natural-sugar content, white crystals may form on the outside over time. Just cover them with a wet towel and the crystals will melt away.

Blissful Fun

Blissful fun recipes are just for fun. We need to have fun when we are alive and well! These shakes are in a category of their own because they are inspired by delicious favorites that create joy in the body. Who doesn't love a little spice in life, some jolt of satisfaction, or an unusually delicious treat—just for fun?

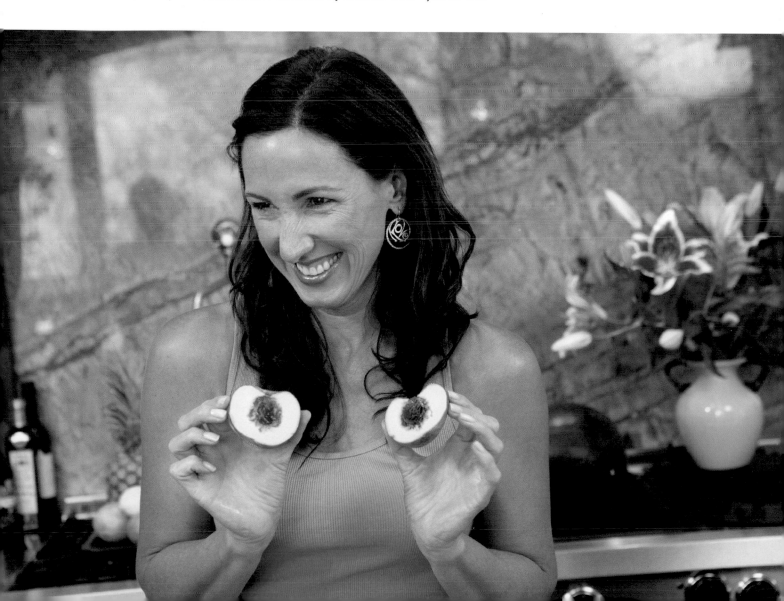

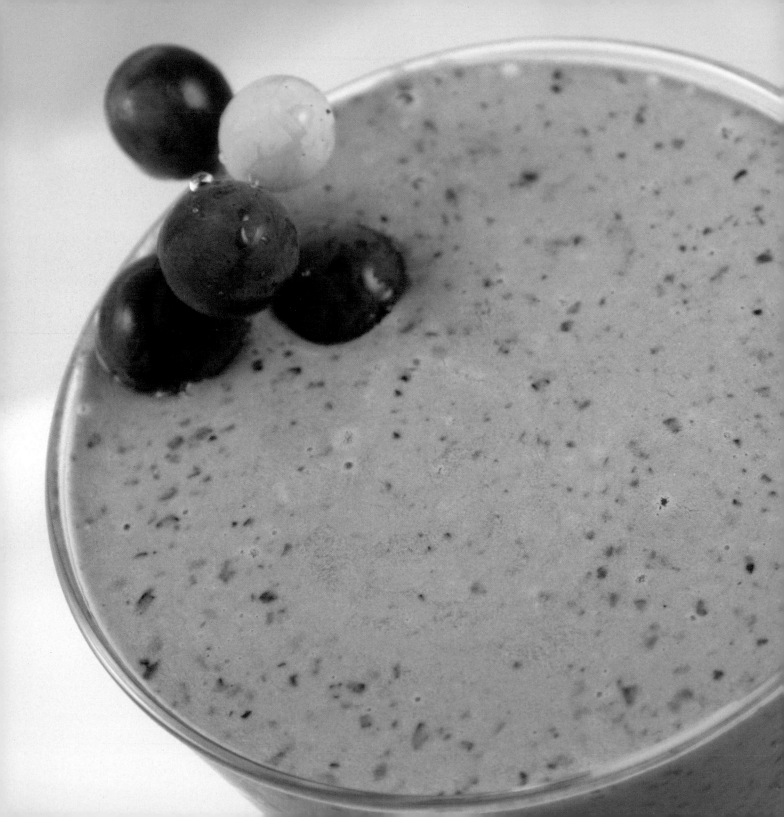

Grape-Ape Chip

Makes 1–2 servings • Prep time: Less than 5 minutes

I have Concord grapevines in my yard that I planted just for fun. They give off a beautiful fruit that tastes just like the old grape juice I drunk as a child. You can find the rich purple, tart, and slightly sweet fruit in markets in late September to October. Using grapes with seeds gives you the extra powered nutrients of the seed energy in this delicious, creamy-yet-tangy grape shake.

Ingredients
1 cup Coconut Bliss Vanilla Island

2 cups organic Concord grapes with seeds

Directions
Blend all ingredients on high until smooth and creamy.

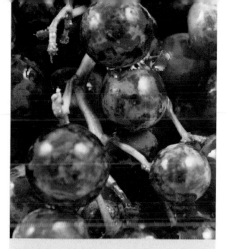

FUN FACT: Eating too many grapes can have a laxative effect.

NUTRITIONAL BENEFIT: Grapes contain caffeic acid, which is a strong cancer-fighting substance.

HOW TO SELECT: Choose organic, in season, and with seeds.

Grape seeds contain resveratrol, flavonoids, and tannin, which are excellent antioxidants.

Green Tea, Please

Makes 1–2 servings • Prep time: Less than 5 minutes

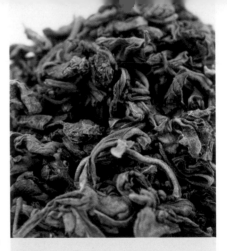

This shake has a certain style and elegance to it. I always feel as if I am in a specialty tea shop when enjoying this "green tea latte." There are different kinds of green tea, each with its own specific flavor and antioxidant compound; I would choose a favorite or two and mix them up. This one must be served in a pretty glass.

Ingredients

    1 cup Coconut Bliss Vanilla Island

    1 cup green tea, brewed and chilled

    1 teaspoon raw honey

    1 cup of ice (optional)

Directions

Brew the tea and add the honey while it's still hot so it dissolves in the tea. Let cool, add to blender with Bliss, and blend on high until smooth and creamy.

FUN FACT: Green tea is green because it is not fermented.

NUTRITIONAL BENEFIT: Green tea contains natural flouride, which is a known cavity fighter.

HOW TO SELECT: Buy organic green tea and store your tea in a dark, dry place.

Green, black, and oolong teas contain potent antioxidants known as polyphenols, but green tea contains the most potent form.

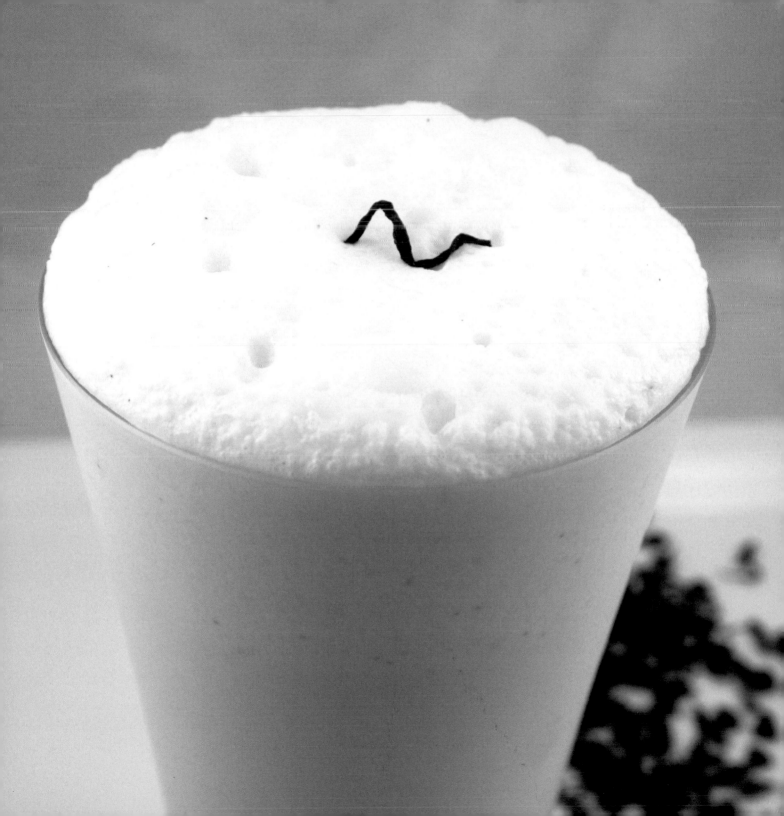

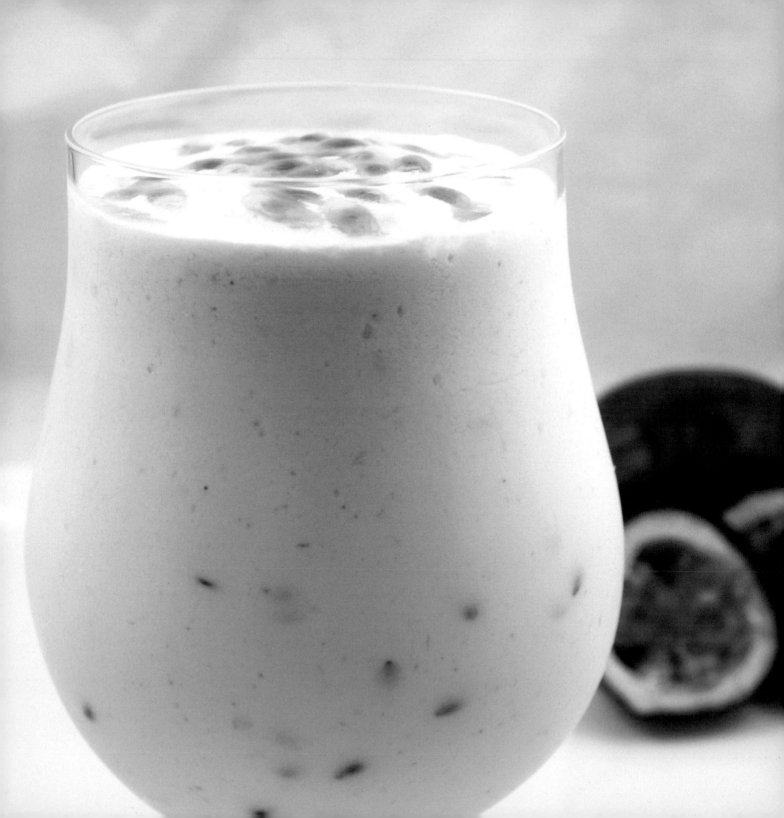

Passionate Kisses

Makes 1–2 servings • Prep time: Less than 5 minutes

Passion fruit is one of the most delicious fruits. They are hard to find unless you live in the tropics. I have recently discovered a passion fruit farm in California that delivers to a local natural foods store, and I buy up what I can, then freeze the puree for future fun. This shake is slightly tart and very refreshing. It makes my mouth water just thinking about it.

Ingredients

1½ cups Coconut Bliss Vanilla Island

½ cup coconut water

2 tablespoons passion fruit pulp (about 2 passion fruits)

Directions

Cut fresh passion fruit in half and scoop out seeded pulp. Blend all ingredients on high until smooth and creamy.

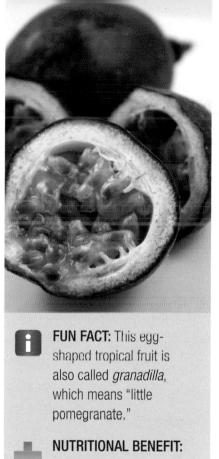

FUN FACT: This egg-shaped tropical fruit is also called *granadilla*, which means "little pomegranate."

NUTRITIONAL BENEFIT: Passion fruit is a beautifying fruit with its high content of vitamin A.

HOW TO SELECT: Choose large, heavy, firm fruit. When ripe, it has wrinkled, dimpled, deep purple skin.

The seeds of the passion fruit contain a relaxing substance that can cause overall calm.

Get Figgy With It

Makes 1–2 servings • Prep time: Less than 5 minutes

Originally this was going to be a vanilla and fig shake, and then I got this hit that black figs and chocolate can be so decadent together that I just had to try it. It is mind-boggling good. You can still make this with vanilla and I'm sure it will be beautiful, but once you go dark chocolate, you may never go back.

Ingredients

> 1½ cups Coconut Bliss Dark Chocolate
>
> ½ cup coconut water
>
> 5–6 dried black figs, soaked
>
> Water for soaking (reserve ½ cup)

Directions

Soak figs for about an hour to soften. Pour them into the blender with ½ cup of the soaking water, add coconut water and Bliss, and blend on high until smooth and creamy.

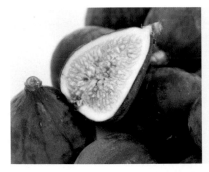

 FUN FACT: Figs are actually a flower inverted into itself, even though they are considered a fruit.

 NUTRITIONAL BENEFIT: Of all common fresh fruits, figs have the most mineral content.

 HOW TO SELECT: Choose figs that are soft but not mushy.

Figs are beautifying and are also said to have aphrodisiac qualities.

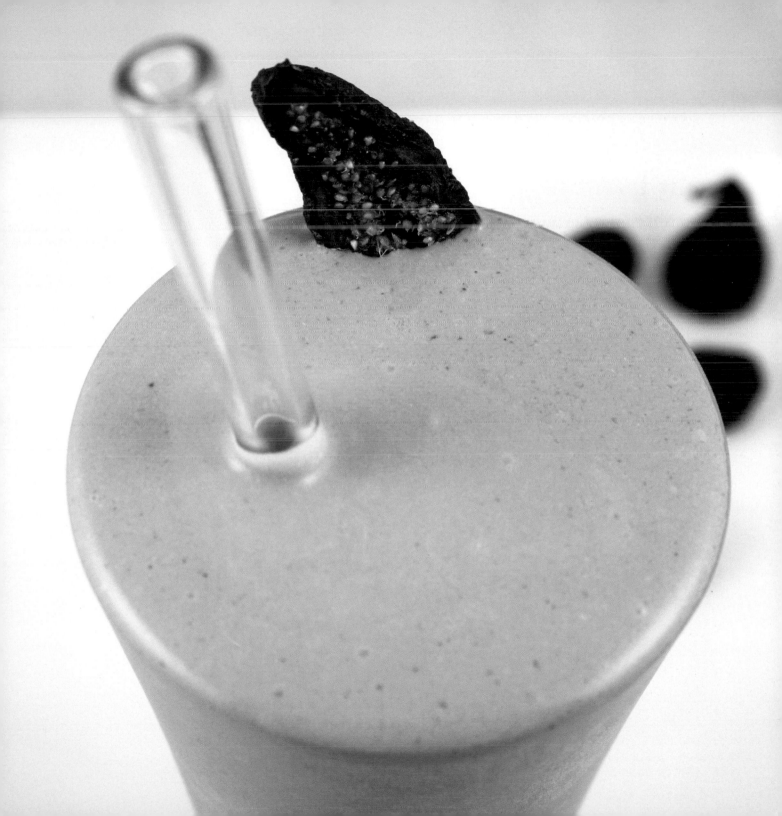

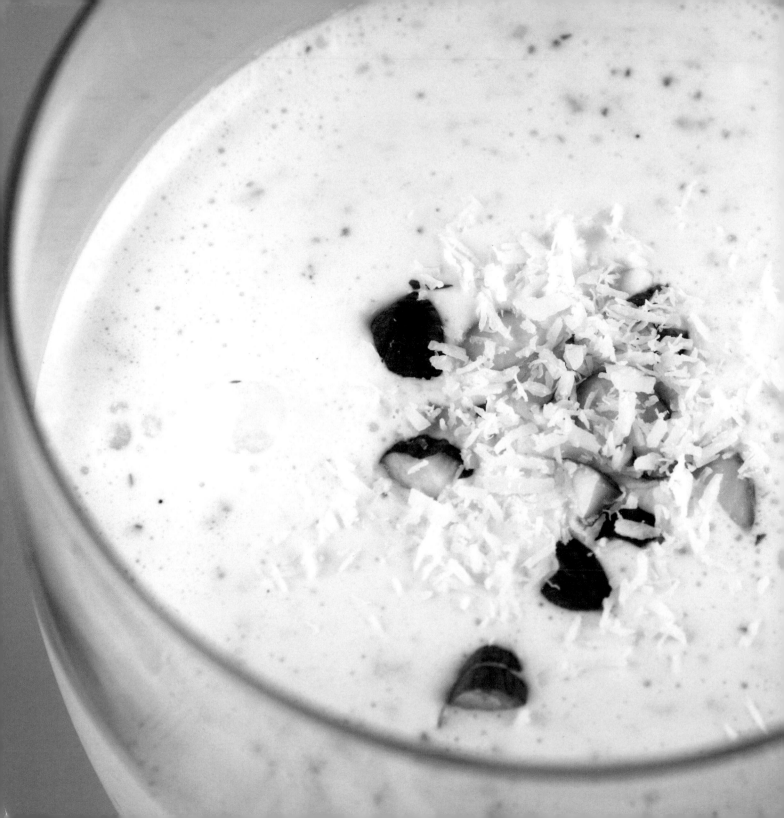

Coco Nutty

Makes 1–2 servings • Prep time: Less than 5 minutes

I made this for my family thinking it was a simple recipe that would go unnoticed, but it turned out to be a huge hit. Coconut is a staple in our house: coconut milk, coconut water, Coconut Bliss, and Coco Nutty non-dairy milkshakes. If you are crazy for coconut or like to chew your shake, you will love this. It's like the ultimate coconut experience.

Ingredients

1½ cups Coconut Bliss Naked Coconut or Vanilla Island

1 cup coconut milk

¼ cup raw unsweetened shredded coconut

¼ cup fresh raw almonds

Directions

Blend all coconut ingredients on high until smooth and creamy. Add almonds and pulse until desired nuttiness.

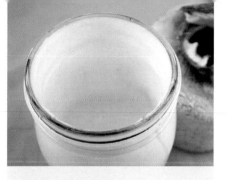

Coconut Milk

Makes about 2 cups • Prep time: From a few minutes if using fresh frozen coconut meat to however long it takes you to crack the coconut yourself

Preparing coconut milk is easy, but opening the coconut is an acquired skill. Practice and diligence make for expert fun. If you are lucky, you can find fresh frozen coconut meat and water at your local grocer (see pp. 24 and 25 for a few brand suggestions).

Ingredients

1 cup coconut meat from a young Thai coconut

1 cup coconut water from a young Thai coconut

Directions

Blend and enjoy! Stays fresh in refrigerator for up to 5 days.

Spice It Up

Makes 1–2 servings • Prep time: Less than 5 minutes

I like my chai spicy and rich, but I am a bit conservative on this recipe. I believe it's easier to add the flavors that excite you rather than subtract. So feel free to adjust the ingredients and spice it up, making your chai spice the way you like it.

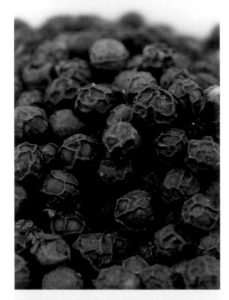

Ingredients

1 cup Coconut Bliss Vanilla Island

1 cup brewed and chilled black tea

¼ teaspoon ground cardamom

¼ teaspoon ground ginger

¼ teaspoon ground cinnamon

⅛ teaspoon ground cloves

⅛ teaspoon ground black pepper

2 Medjool dates, pitted

1 cup ice cubes

Directions

Blend all ingredients on high until smooth and creamy.

 FUN FACT: Black pepper contains piperine, which stimulates the nerve endings in your mucus membranes, causing you to sneeze.

NUTRITIONAL BENEFIT: Black pepper stimulates the breakdown of fat cells while giving you energy to burn.

 HOW TO SELECT: Choose dark black peppercorns and freshly grind them when possible.

If you are feeling like being uncomplicated today, you may brew your favorite chai tea, sweeten with honey, chill, and blend with Bliss and ice for a frozen "chai latte."

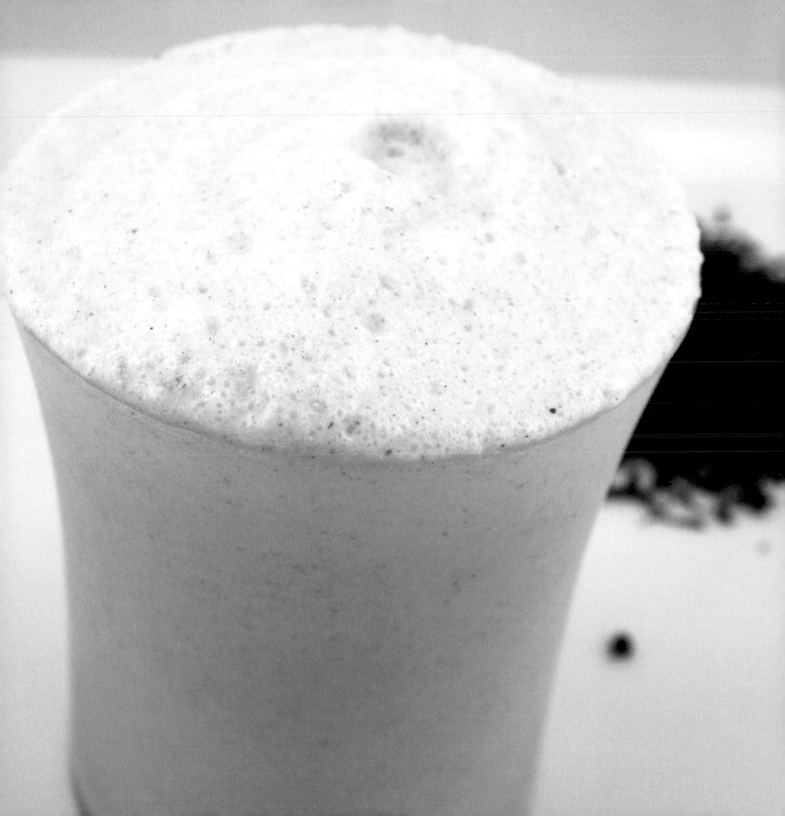

Wanna Date Me?

Makes 1–2 servings • Prep time: Less than 5 minutes

This shake is cute and simple, but certainly no wallflower. It is a simple delight to enjoy anytime, anywhere. If you want to add a bit of adventure and mystery to this basic date shake, then throw in some beet greens or spinach and some fresh fruit or berries—you may find that this is the best date you ever had.

Ingredients

1 cup Coconut Bliss Vanilla Island

1 cup almond milk (or nut or seed milk of choice)

¼ cup Medjool dates, pitted

Directions

Blend all ingredients on high until smooth and creamy.

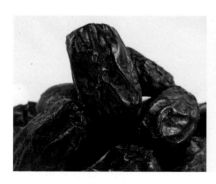

 FUN FACT: Dates are the sweetest fruit.

 NUTRITIONAL BENEFIT: Dates contain more potassium than bananas and provide instant energy.

 HOW TO SELECT: Look for moist, plump dates.

Dates are rich in iron and can be eaten on a daily basis.

Driving Me Bananas

Makes 1–2 servings • Prep time: Less than 5 minutes

By now, you should have a big bag of frozen bananas in your freezer waiting for a smoothie to happen. If you're anything like me, you have two to three bags and they are driving you bananas taking up all that space. Time to whip up a delicious and easy milkshake for friends. Serve it for dessert in a beautiful glass, add some caramel sauce (see p. 130), and you have a show stopper.

Ingredients
- 1 cup Coconut Bliss Vanilla Island
- 1 cup almond milk (or nut or seed milk of choice)
- 1 frozen banana

Directions
Blend all ingredients on high until smooth and creamy.

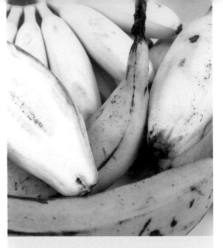

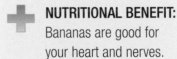

FUN FACT: A cluster of bananas is called a hand. A hand consists of 10 to 20 bananas, which are known as fingers.

NUTRITIONAL BENEFIT: Bananas are good for your heart and nerves.

HOW TO SELECT: A ripe banana is sweeter because the starch turns to sugar.

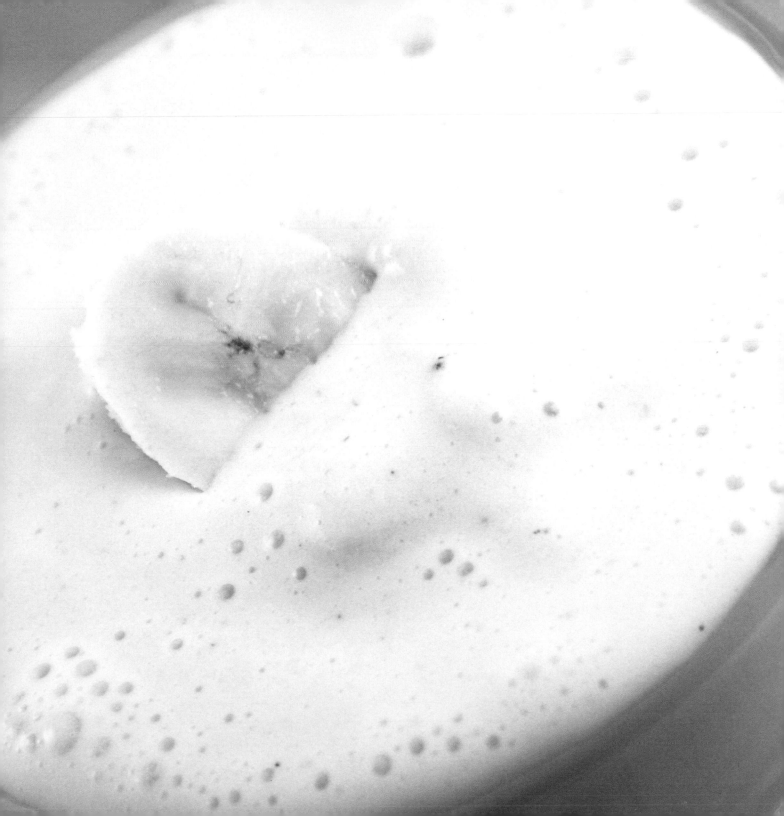

Diana's Walk-Away Message

I can honestly say that I am an expert in ME. I am not a doctor, a scientist, or even a certified nutritionist. I am a woman who has healed herself through food. I have a lifetime of experience and knowledge about the effects of food on the body, and the one thing I know is that we are all unique beings with different needs and values. What I want most of all is for each of you to become an expert in your own body. Find and know the things that work for you. I fully recognize that what I write to you may not work for everyone. I encourage you to experiment and explore, to make substitutions that make your life blissful.

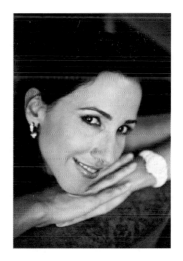

I have had so much fun creating recipes for you. I wanted to work with products like Coconut Bliss to make it easier for each of us to get maximum taste along with health benefits. I am aware that these products are not available everywhere, and it may cause some disruption in your quest for Bliss. Feel free to find a local product with equal simplicity and flavor, or simply make your own non-dairy ice creams—whatever brings overall joy and bliss to your Naked lifestyle. Learning to prepare your own food will definitely ensure a healthier life as we can never be quite sure what we are getting when we place food preparation into the hands of others.

Next time you are out and about and you crave something along the lines of a Naked Bliss shake, remember that the shakes from the coffee house on the street corner or in the mall are simply an empty, quick fix for the desire for real food. Perhaps the next time you see someone drinking an oversized fruit smoothie that contains sherbet, sweet and syrupy frozen fruit, and so-called "boosters," you will remember how lucky you are to know the difference between hype and really good nutrition. I am always comforted in knowing that there is no deprivation in a Naked lifestyle, only good sense, good nutrition, and flavorful treats that make you feel so good.

I made a promise in *Get Naked Fast! A Guide to Stripping Away the Foods That Weigh You Down* to continue providing loving and delicious recipes to keep you on your path to wellness. I hope that *Naked Bliss* gives you some fun options to keep you satisfied.

In health and love,

-Diana

Recipe Index

Almond Milk, 27

Apple Pie & Ice Cream, 84

Bee My Honey, 108

Beet It, 77

Blackberry Bliss, 54

Blissful Nog, 91

Blueberry Bliss, 61

Café Crème, 92

Caramel Apple, 88

Caramel Sauce, 88, 130

Cherry Vanilla Chocolate Chip, 126

Chocolate-Covered Banana, 137

Chocolate Orange Chip, 133

Coconut Almond Fudge, 138

Coconut Milk, 151

Coco Nutty, 151

Cold-Pressed Coffee, 92

Cool as a Cucumber, 69

Cran-Apple, 50

Cranberry Chip, 112

Creamsicle Bliss, 111

Creamy Caramel Swirl, 130

Double Chocolate Chip, 99

Driving Me Bananas, 156

French Vanilla, 96

Fudge Drizzle, 138

Garden Bliss, 65

Get Figgy With It, 148

Goji Mojo, 104

Goji Mojo Chip, 104

Grape-Ape Chip, 143

Green Tea, Please, 144

Just Plum Good, 46

Kale Colada, 74

Lettuce C, 66

Lettuce Sea U Smile, 78

Mango Lassi, 57

Mango Raspberry Bliss, 58

Mint Chocolate Chip, 119

Minty Fudge, 125

Mocha Almond Fudge, 129

New York Cheesecake, 100

Papaya Lemongrass, 49

Passionate Kisses, 147

Popeye's Cream Dream, 70

Pumpkin Pie Spice, 87

Rainbow Cream, 73

Red Velvet, 134

Rejuvelac, 39

Southern Comfort, 115

Spice It Up, 152

Strawberry Cream, 95

Strawberry Peach Daiquiri, 45

Strawberry Recharge, 107

Sweet Cherry Love, 116

Sweet Pea, 81

Tropical Bliss, 53

Vanilla Malted, 120

Wanna Date Me?, 155

About the Author

Diana Stobo is a successful Mill Valley, California, based raw-food expert. She is a culinary artist and raw-food advocate who has created delicious and fully accessible recipes that help maintain the Naked Nourishment lifestyle. She is the author of the rapidly selling book, *Get Naked Fast! A Guide to Stripping Away the Foods That Weigh You Down.* Diana is living proof that her Naked Nourishment lifestyle works.

Once plagued by relentless pain and physical discomfort caused by food toxicity, Diana successfully navigated her way through old patterns to discover a healthy way of eating and living. She has transformed her life into one of optimal health, vibrance, and beauty. Passionate about everything in life including her relationships, family, wellness, and especially her food, Diana understands how integral food is to all aspects of nutrition including child development, family patterns, social expectations, and body awareness.

As someone who looks and feels younger than she did 10 years ago, Diana's philosophy is to empower yourself with food choices that give you a better lifestyle. Diana's goal is to design nutritious, accessible products—familiar foods with taste and flare—while introducing exciting and healthful new ingredients. Diana integrates the whole of her experience, including her early teenage tart-baking business, training in Cornell University's School of Hotel Administration culinary arts division, and running her highly successful Signature Catering business.

Diana regularly conducts instructional sessions at major and local natural food markets, farmers' markets, wellness festivals, spas, medical and health facilities, and corporations that educate customers on the advantages of a raw-food lifestyle.

Combining professional expertise with rich personal experience, Diana is dedicated to creating delicious, nutritious recipes that are easy to prepare and satisfying to the senses. Feasting while dropping excess weight, increasing physical and mental energy, and staying young and sexy while developing a healthier relationship with food—this is the Naked Nourishment lifestyle that Diana has discovered for herself and wishes to share with you!